SHIFT56

GW00731834

THE SHIFT56 SYSTEM

By Jon Lipsey, Joe Warner and Josh Cuthbert
Contributing Editors Tom Eastham, Kim Ingleby, Krista Scott-Dixon,
Brian St Pierre, Kimberley Wilson

Creative Director	Ash Gibson
Photography Director	Glen Burrows
Model	Jaimie-Beth Geraghty
Stylist	Lee Holden
Managing Editor	Chris Miller
Additional Photography	Getty, iStock

ISBN 978-1-9998728-0-9
Copyright © IronLife Media Ltd 2017

While every care was taken during the production of this book, the publisher cannot be held responsible for the accuracy of the information or any consequence arising from it. The health, fitness and nutrition information presented in this book is intended as an educational resource and is not intended as a substitute for medical advice. Before starting any exercise programme you should consider consulting a qualified fitness professional to ensure the regime is suitable for you, and your own doctor, especially if you have a medical condition, are taking medication or have related concerns. Discontinue any exercise that causes you pain or severe discomfort and consult a medical expert. The publisher cannot be held responsible for any injuries which may occur as a result of these exercises. The publisher is not liable for the contents of any external internet sites listed or linked to, nor does it endorse any commercial product or service mentioned or advised on any of the sites.

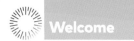
Contents

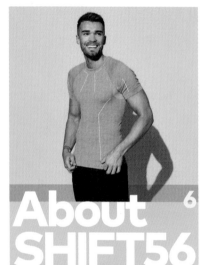

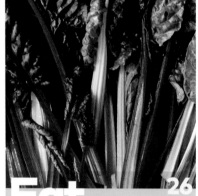

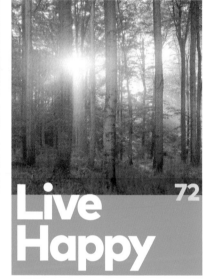

About SHIFT56 — 6

Eat Smart — 26

Live Happy — 72

Ready to live a healthier and happier life?
Here's what you'll find in the six sections of
The SHIFT56 System to help you do just that!

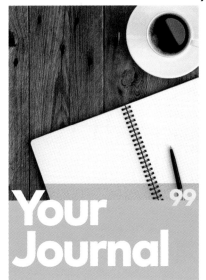

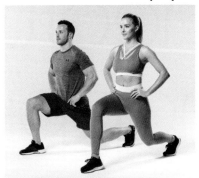

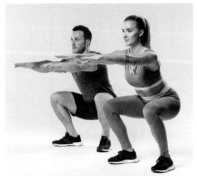

Your Journal 99

Train Smart 187

Form Guides 222

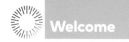

Your healthier and happier life starts now!

Welcome to The SHIFT56 System, your complete guide to a healthier and happier life!

Hi, and welcome to The SHIFT56 System! You're holding this book in your hands for a very simple reason: you want to make some really positive – and lasting – changes to the way you look and feel.

Maybe you've attempted to become healthier and happier before by following an exercise and eating plan – perhaps one with an attention-grabbing name – that promised to turn your life around immediately. But it didn't work, and that's why you're reading this now.

Don't worry: you are not alone! The unfortunate truth is that most people who try to become fitter and healthier fail to change, even if they start with sky-high levels of motivation.

But the days of disappointment and frustration are over. Because there's a reason you haven't achieved your health and happiness goals (yet) – and it's not your fault!

The real reason
The reason is not that you failed. Maybe it felt that way, but it's important you realise *you* weren't the reason you didn't make the positive changes you wanted. It was because of the flaws in the plan you were following.

Let this sink in. You didn't fail that plan; that plan failed you. Its too-good-to-be-true promise was exactly that – too good to be true!

Perhaps the exercise plan was too intense, with hours of exercise every day. Or the diet was so strict and short of nutrients that you looked and felt terrible. Maybe it was a combination of the two: intense workouts on a disastrous – and dangerous – diet that claimed you'd lose loads of weight in an impossibly short time.

I know plans like that – and I hate them. They drain away your positivity and after only a few days your motivation, willpower and confidence have been replaced by fatigue, misery and hunger. So much for that promise of a healthier and happier life!

There is a better way!
Living a leaner, healthier and happier life is achievable for everyone – including you – but only if you take the smart approach. And that's what The SHIFT56 System is. It will guide you towards greater – and lasting – health and happiness, starting right now!

The SHIFT56 System has been designed by top experts to empower you to make small and sustainable exercise, eating and lifestyle changes over the next 56 days – changes that quickly add up so that in just eight weeks you will look and feel healthier and happier than you ever thought possible.

And I know this plan works. How? Because I've already done it! And so has my celebrity co-author Josh Cuthbert! Turn the page to discover how The SHIFT56 System helped Josh become leaner, healthier and happier than ever.

Then the best bit begins: it's your turn to change your life for the better! Ready? Let's do this!

Joe Warner,
Editor

Remember: go to shift56.com to sign up for our brilliant – and free – health and happiness newsletters!

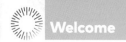
'I want you to be as happy as I am!'

Here's how Josh Cuthbert got on following The SHIFT56 System, and what you can expect

Josh Cuthbert is a busy man. As well as recording with his band Union J, he's a model for some of the fashion world's most prestigious brands, a radio presenter and an Instagram influencer with hundreds of thousands of followers. But by following The SHIFT56 System Josh found it easier than he ever thought possible to become healthier and happier, despite his hectic schedule. Here he shares his insights from following The SHIFT56 System and reveals what you can expect from the plan that will make you leaner, healthier and happier than ever before!

What did you like about the SHIFT56 exercise plan?
The workouts are easy to understand and easy to follow, but still challenging enough for me to notice positive changes straight away. Because all the exercises in the plan are bodyweight moves I didn't need any kit or equipment so I could do the sessions at home or wherever I was, which is really good when I'm out on the road working. There was no excuse not to find half an hour to do a workout, and I always felt so much better for doing them! I actually did a lot of the plan's workouts with my fiancée [model Chloe Lloyd] – doing it with someone else was great and we could push and motivate each other. And it felt great that we were both getting leaner and stronger together. You feel more fit, lean and confident with each passing week.

How did you fit the exercise plan into your busy life?
I did my sessions on Mondays, Wednesdays and Fridays, first thing in the morning. It was great to exercise first thing and then feel a lot more energised for the rest of the day. It was a bit tough at first – well, starting any new habit is – but we soon got into our new routine and even started looking forward to the next workout because we got such a buzz from doing them. Chloe was new to exercise, but because of the way the plan

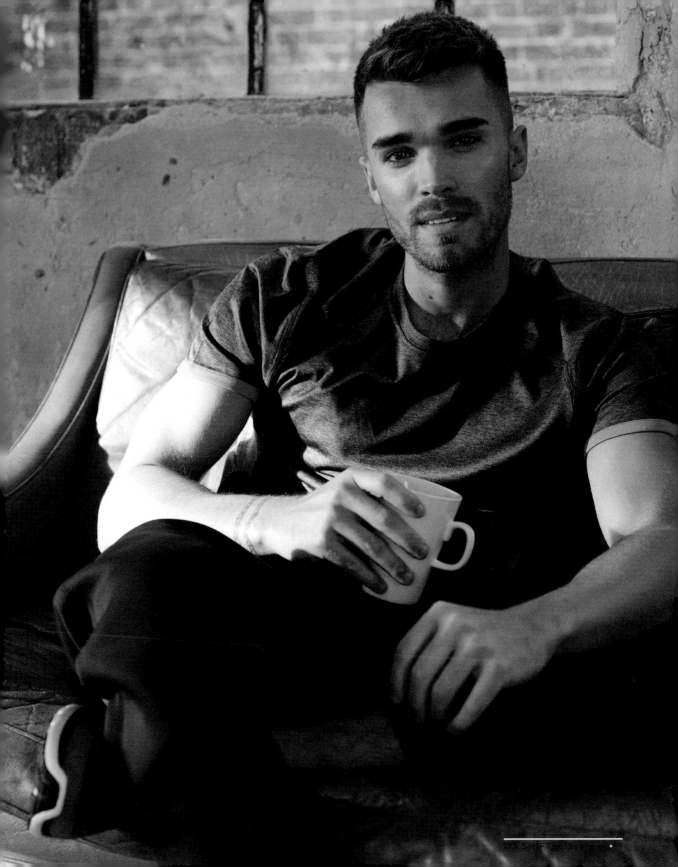

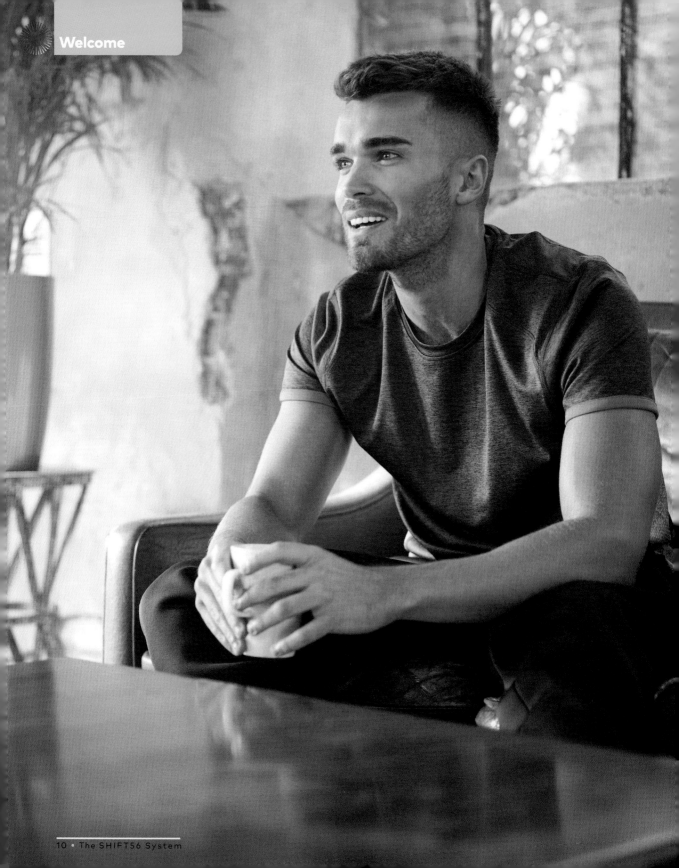

works, we could still do it together and that was great. We motivated each other and when one of us was finding it tough, the other one could offer some encouragement. Training together meant we both pushed harder than we would have done alone – it was healthy competition, shall I say...

What surprised you most about the exercise plan?
Exercise is obviously really important for being fitter and healthier, and it's one of the best ways to lose weight – and keep it off – but we also noticed lots of mental benefits, which are just as important. Exercise is the ultimate stress-buster and I always felt great finishing a session – positive, motivated and happy! If you feel positive it makes each training session much more enjoyable... well, it makes *everything* more enjoyable. I can't imagine not having exercise as a part of my life now. It's "me time" where I put my health and happiness first.

What did you like most about the SHIFT56 eating plan?
The plan is based on eating well 80% of the time, which means that for the other 20% we could still eat all the foods we love, without feeling bad or guilty about it. The approach gives me the flexibility to eat for better health most of the time, but without all that pressure and misery of giving up certain foods or entire food groups, which happens on most quick-fix diets! It accommodates holidays, parties, all social occasions – we never feel stressed or worried about what we can and can't eat. And it gives us total freedom to eat well and eat the foods we love! We tend to eat very healthily Monday to Friday and then let loose a little bit more during weekends!

So you still eat all the foods you love?
Absolutely! I love my food, so this is very important – I never feel like I am depriving myself. The SHIFT56 approach is about installing some balance into our diets, so we eat the right foods for better health most of the time, but we can always eat meals or snacks purely for pleasure when we want. It's the best of both worlds, and I never thought eating this well would be this easy!

How much easier do you find it now to eat better and more mindfully?
Eating more mindfully is something I'd never really thought about – when you're busy it's so tempting to just wolf down food without even thinking about what or how much you're eating! Eating mindfully has been a revelation and has transformed my relationship with food for the better. It's so easy too – it can be as simple as Chloe and me eating together at the table and not in front of the TV, or taking a few moments to look at and smell the meal before we start eating. It's taught me how to eat until I'm satisfied, not until I'm stuffed. That makes a big difference to how I feel and means I don't eat more than I need. There's nothing wrong with leaving the odd piece of food on your plate. Eating together without distraction has other benefits – we talk more about our days and other things going on, which helps me deal with the stress of daily life. I can't believe how effective it is and I just wish I'd started doing it sooner!

How did you get on with The SHIFT56 System's journal?
I really love the journal! It's brilliant to get thoughts and feelings out of my head, where they can be overwhelming, and into my journal, so I could take a step back from them and not get too stressed. It's so easy to do and it doesn't take very long – but it's so helpful! I can't believe what a difference it's made to so many different parts of my life. I never thought the simple act of writing things down could have such a massive positive impact. I feel less stressed and more in control, and it makes finding the time to eat well and exercise so much easier. I can't emphasise it enough – this journal is life-changing! I just wish I'd done something like this years ago.

What did you like most about the journal?
It only takes a few minutes a day, so no time at all really, but the simple act of writing down a few things – how I am feeling, what I am grateful for, what I want to achieve today or this week – allowed me to really quickly and simply take a step back and get some perspective on my life. And when you have that perspective it makes it so much easier to see what I need to do more of, or less of, and then put that thought into practice! I see my journal as "me time" each day to focus on me and what I want in life. It's really important to spend a little time each day just to focus on yourself and living the life you want. When you think like this it becomes easy to find the time to do your journal – in many ways it's the most important time of my day.

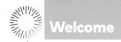

The SHIFT56 Squad

Here is the team behind The SHIFT56 System

JOSH CUTHBERT

Josh is a singer in the band Union J, which formed during the ninth season of *The X Factor*. He is also a model and has worked with brands including Dolce & Gabbana, Paco Rabanne and Next, as well as having his own show on Heat Radio on Sundays between midday and 2pm.

My favourite meal is...
Japanese cuisine! I'm a big fan of gyozas, chicken katsu, noodles and sushi.

I love exercise because...
It makes me feel good. I like setting myself a challenge and a target to achieve. It's also great to know that exercise makes my body leaner, fitter and healthier, and also makes me more positive, motivated, confident and ultimately happier!

I am at my happiest when...
I'm sat on the sofa with my fiancée Chloe watching an amazing Netflix series after a great workout – because if I've just done a good workout, I don't feel bad for slouching on the sofa!

JOE WARNER

Joe is a bestselling fitness author, and a regular expert contributor to the BBC and other national and international media.

My favourite meal is...
Does a bowl of banana ice cream count as a meal? What about a cheese board? OK, then I'll go for a home-made lasagne and a (big) glass of good red. Followed by banana ice cream or a cheese board.

I love exercise because...
It lets me work up a sweat and blow off some steam, and it allows me to take a break from everyday stresses and get some perspective. Humans are made to move, and spending too long sitting down isn't good for our bodies or our brains!

I am at my happiest when...
Running on a beach (somewhere hot, preferably) or with my closest friends and family with good food and good music, and without a care in the world.

JON LIPSEY

Jon is an award-winning fitness writer and the most successful ever editor of *Men's Fitness* magazine. He has worked as a health and well-being expert for some of the world's biggest brands and is a regular speaker at fitness conventions.

My favourite meal is...
A big spicy brunch of Mexican-style baked eggs with avocado. Add a generous cup of good-quality coffee and I'm a happy man. And if Joe's willing to share his ice cream, I'll have a bowl of that too.

I love exercise because...
It makes me feel more energised. Maybe not when I'm lying in a pool of sweat at the end of a tough workout, but in life generally!

I am at my happiest when...
I'm outdoors having an adventure in a beautiful part of the world, or when I'm sharing a bottle of wine and a joke with family and friends.

KIMBERLEY WILSON

Kimberley is a chartered psychologist and founder of Monumental Health, a London clinic dedicated to addressing the psychological, physiological and lifestyle drivers of mental illness. Her integrated service uses evidence-based nutritional and lifestyle interventions, alongside psychological therapy, to provide a complete and personalised approach to mental healthcare.

My favourite meal is...
A tough call between spaghetti and meatballs and a good burrito. Or ramen. I love all the food!

I love exercise because...
It makes you smarter, stronger, healthier, happier, resilient... and lots more!

I am at my happiest when...
I'm grateful. Corny but true.

KIM INGLEBY

Kim is a multiple award-winning mind and body expert who is passionate about helping people let go of their fears and unlock their full potential. She is a TEDx speaker and the author of *Hound Of Happiness: 52 Tips To Feel Good*.

My favourite meal is...

A chicken stir-fry with fresh oregano, chilli, garlic, ginger and lime, with mushrooms, asparagus, courgettes, broccoli, sun-dried tomatoes and black olives.

I love exercise because...

I love seeing what's possible with my body, learning, adapting and becoming stronger. Training gives me headspace and grows my confidence, improves my posture, boosts my immunity and helps my sleep.

I am at my happiest when...

I'm wandering in the wild countryside, mountains or sea, with my family and my own "Hound of Happiness" Jake.

 KRISTA SCOTT DIXON

Krista taught and researched at York University in Toronto for ten years before joining Precision Nutrition as director of curriculum. She's the editor of the PN Level 1 textbook *The Essentials of Sport & Exercise Nutrition* and the author of *Genetics: The Universe Within*.

My favourite meal is...

A big, sweaty plate of barbecue brisket or ribs.

I love exercise because...

I don't have a choice – exercise is life! Movement is a way for humans to express themselves and be in the world. When we stop moving, we start decaying.

I am at my happiest when...

I'm anywhere nature is large and in charge!

 TOM EASTHAM

Tom is a personal trainer who works with clients ranging from professional rugby players and MMA fighters to everyday gym-goers. He also consults for brands, including Technogym and PowerPlate, on making elite-level training methods more accessible to the masses.

My favourite meal is...

Roast beef, Yorkshire puddings and all the trimmings!

I love exercise because...

Exercise is a fundamental part of being a human being. I firmly believe that you have a right to see the full beauty of what your body is capable of. Training is my opportunity to push myself mentally and physically to the limits of my capability to fulfil my potential.

I am at my happiest when...

I'm in the kitchen, cooking a meal for friends, or walking my dogs in a park or forest far away from city life.

 BRIAN ST PIERRE

Brian is the director of performance nutrition at Precision Nutrition, coaching elite athletes and working with professional sports teams. Brian has authored several books, including *The High Performance Handbook: Nutrition Guide*. He holds a master's degree in food science and human nutrition and is a registered dietitian.

My favourite meal is...

An English muffin with peanut butter. I could eat melted peanut butter all day!

I love exercise because...

It gives me energy and strength to play with my kids, enjoy outdoor activities, do my job and feel confident. It improves my health, helps me manage stress and sleep well, and has a positive impact on every area of my life.

I am at my happiest when...

I am playing outside with my wife and children. I love my job and I love getting things done, but most of all I love getting to experience again the carefree play of children.

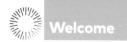

Your quick-

Start living a healthier and happier life today!

We recommend you read the whole of this book in order to really understand how and why this plan will make you healthier and happier than ever. But if you're short of time or super-keen to get your SHIFT56 journey started, here's what to do!

1 Move your body!

Raring to go? Great! You can find your first exercise session on p190, and the instructions to start the plan quickly and effectively. The best bit – aside from that it's going to help you shift body fat really fast – is that you don't need any specialist equipment, so you can do your sessions any time, anywhere. Just make some space and start working up a sweat!

start guide

2 Start eating smarter!

If you're like us, you love your food. And the beauty of our smarter eating plan is you don't have to give up your favourite foods, go hungry or count calories! Our super-easy Perfect Portion approach to healthier eating starts on p52, and check out our quick guide on how to be more mindful during meals on p64. Why? It's the easiest yet most beneficial thing you can do to look and feel better today!

3 Set your goal!

We want you to be happier – it's why we made this book! On p90 you'll discover how to select the perfect eight-week health and happiness goal for you to start working towards. Don't worry if the thought of choosing a goal feels daunting or difficult right now – we've got a fantastic and fun exercise to make picking your goal exciting and empowering!

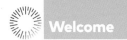

The SHIFT56 System: how the plan works

We want you to be healthier and happier – it's why we made this book!

The way to become truly happy – and we mean not just for a few days or weeks, but for life – is to make small and sustainable steps in the right direction. Before long those simple yet hugely influential lifestyle changes will quickly add up to make you healthier and happier than you ever thought possible.

Trying to overhaul every part of your whole life at the same time and turn every single bad habit into a good one overnight is the biggest mistake people make when wanting to become fitter, healthier and happier. Trying to do too much too soon, all at once, is a recipe for disaster – in fact, it's likely to make you far unhealthier and unhappier.

The beauty of The SHIFT56 System is its simplicity – and you can start right this minute!

The three parts of the plan
The SHIFT56 System is based on three of the most important factors behind achieving greater health and happiness: exercise, eating and journaling. Again, don't worry if you've never exercised before, or kept a journal (which is simply a slightly more structured way of keeping a daily diary). We'll explain everything you need to know and we've made all three elements of this book incredibly easy to follow and understand.

As you will see, the three elements of The SHIFT56 System are all closely linked and interconnected – doing one part makes you more likely and better able to do the others. Think of it as a "virtuous circle" like the one shown on the opposite page.

On the following pages we explain how and why your new eight-week fat loss exercise plan works, then detail how to put your new flexible eating for life approach into practice, and then finally reveal how your new daily journal works to help you achieve your health and happiness goals over the next 56 days.

The SHIFT56 System In Action
The three elements of this book work as a virtuous circle

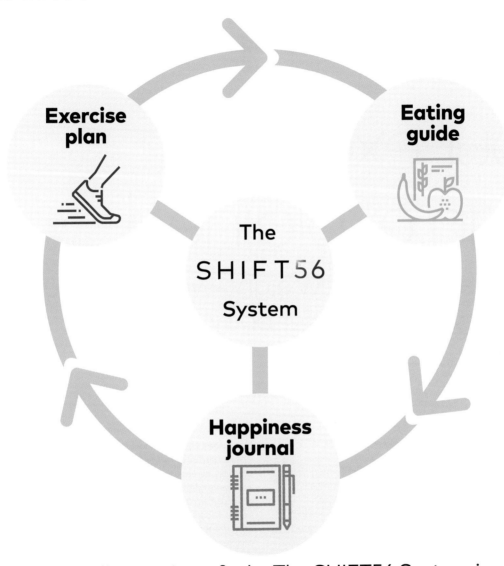

Here's an illustration of why The SHIFT56 System is so effective at helping you become healthier and happier!

- In the morning you do your daily journal entry, which will help you to have a more productive day

- That will ensure you have time to do one of the plan's fat loss workouts, which will make you feel great

- You then eat healthier and more nutritious foods, which gives your body the nutrients it needs to look and feel better

- A productive and less stressful day means you sleep better, so you'll wake up tomorrow full of energy and motivation – so having another successful day is much easier!

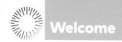

Your exercise plan explained

Here's how your new eight-week workout plan will get you a healthier body and a happier mind!

It's possible to lose weight just through changes to how you eat (we'll get to that next!), but add exercise to the mix and you'll lose fat even faster – and gain many extra physical and mental health benefits to change the way you look and feel for the better.

The best bit? Your SHIFT56 exercise plan couldn't be easier to understand or to follow. You don't need to go to a gym, the workouts don't take long, and you can do them all in the comfort of your own home!

The plan is based on a type of exercise called high-intensity functional training, which research proves is a better way of burning fat and defining muscles than high-intensity interval training (HIIT) or low-intensity steady-state cardio, such as jogging.

We love this type of training so much that the title of this book is an acronym of Smart High-Intensity Functional Training (that explains SHIFT – and 56, of course, is the number of days in the eight-week plan). The full exercise chapter starts on p187, but here's an overview of it – and why it's so great!

How does the plan work?
There are three workouts a week for the next eight weeks, so 24 in total. Each workout is made up of a set number of circuits, in which you do a set number of exercises in order, resting briefly between moves, then return to the start and repeat the circuit. It's that simple!

Do the workouts change?
Each workout is different: the exercises you do, the time you do them for, and how long you rest before the next one all vary from workout to workout. This approach is incredibly effective at burning body fat and defining muscles to transform your body for the better, but it's still straightforward and easy to follow – even if you've never exercised before!

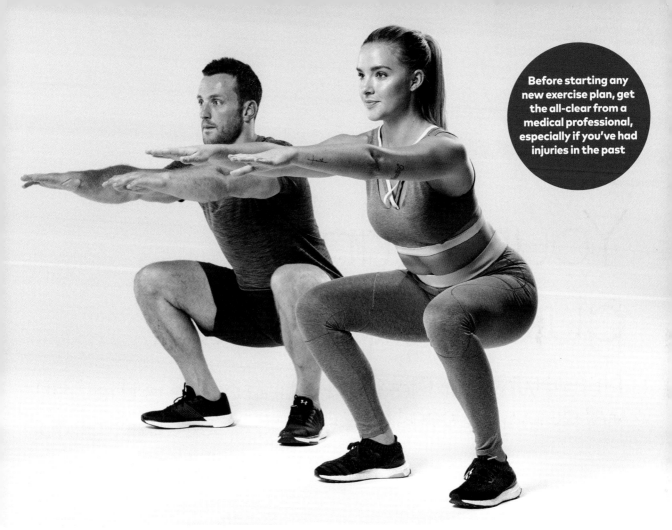

Before starting any new exercise plan, get the all-clear from a medical professional, especially if you've had injuries in the past

What kit or equipment do I need?

The best thing about the plan – after the fact that it'll help you shift body fat really fast – is that you don't need a gym membership or any kit, so you can do your sessions at home. All you need is a little space, some water and a towel (you're going to be working up a thirst and a sweat!) to start burning off that fat.

How long does each session take?

The sessions take between 30 and 40 minutes, so it's really easy to squeeze in three sessions each week even if you're very busy. It's best to leave a day between sessions, so doing your three weekly workouts on a Monday, Wednesday and Friday would be perfect, and leaves your weekends free for other fun and relaxing activities.

I've never done an exercise plan before – can I do this?

Yes! The plan has been designed to deliver great results for everyone – whatever your exercise experience! There's nothing complex – you'll do every move in each circuit for a set amount of time, not for a set number of repetitions (reps). So you simply do the exercise as many times as you can within the time allowed. If you're new to training that number might be quite low at first, but you'll soon see some big positive changes! All the exercises in this plan, as well as your warm-up exercise and warm-down stretches, are clearly demonstrated with photos and form guides from p222.

The benefits of exercise include less body fat, more defined muscles, stronger bones, better sleep and mood, less anxiety, and better brain function – one study found exercise reverses age-related brain volume loss! So it helps you lose fat *and* get healthier, happier and smarter!

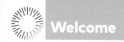
Your eating guide explained

Here's why our Flexible Eating guide is the perfect approach to help you lose fat for good!

What would you think if someone told you that you could lose weight – for good – and still eat all your favourite meals? Too good to be true? Well, we've got some good news for you!

The eating guide in The SHIFT56 System has been designed to help you lose body fat quickly, while not depriving you of your favourite foods nor forcing you to count calories ever again.

Why? Because you don't need to do either of those things to lose weight and then keep it off. There's a far smarter and better way to eat and we think you're going to love it!

Why don't I need to count calories?

Counting calories is a popular approach to losing weight, but it's not that useful. Yes, calories are important because to lose weight you do need to burn off more calories than you eat, but counting calories isn't the smart way to lose fat – because estimating your daily calorie intake and expenditure is almost impossible! We explain why from p34, and then detail why the SHIFT56 Flexible Eating guide is a smarter way to lose fat and keep it off for good!

What is Flexible Eating?

Flexible Eating is so simple yet so brilliant for helping you lose weight. Flexible Eating means you don't need to follow a "perfect" diet 100% of the time, which is not only unsustainable but also encourages an unhealthy relationship with food. The key to losing fat successfully is a consistent approach, and Flexible Eating allows you to eat the foods you love up for up to 20% of your meals. For the other 80% of the time you follow our Perfect Portion approach to meals, which makes eating well easier than you ever thought possible!

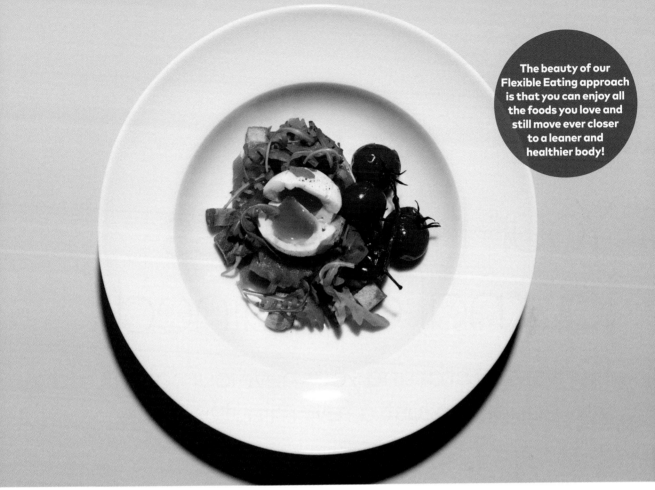

The beauty of our Flexible Eating approach is that you can enjoy all the foods you love and still move ever closer to a leaner and healthier body!

What is the Perfect Portion approach?

It's our smart guide to help you make delicious, nutritious meals without the need for scales or counting calories! Instead you simply use your hand to measure how much protein, carbs, fats and vegetables should make up your meals. The Perfect Portion approach removes all the stress and hassle from eating well for that 80% of the time, and is the best way to eat for better health and happiness without giving up the foods you love. Learn more about the Perfect Portion approach from p50.

Aren't detox diets the best way to lose fat fast?

No, quite the opposite! We explain why on p30. The biggest problem with "detox" and other "quick-fix" diets that promise rapid fat loss is that most of the weight you initially lose is just water. These diets also starve your body of some of the nutrients it needs, which can cause dramatic negative changes throughout your entire body. They also make you more likely to obsess over food and eating, and you're far more likely to regain the weight you've lost – and more besides – when you quit the diet.

What else do I need to know?

The Eat Smart fat loss chapter begins on p26, and there you'll find further explanation of this and much more besides in simple and easy-to-follow terms so you can start eating for a healthier and happier life straight away. One thing you definitely should read is our guide to being Mindful at Mealtimes on p64: it's one of the quickest and easiest things you can do to start losing weight today – and you will be amazed at just how easy it is!

Quick tip

Many people fail to lose weight because they start following a very strict diet plan that's impossible to stick to for long. Any weight they lose they normally regain, along with frustration and unhappiness! Our eating guide is an approach you can follow indefinitely to lose fat without giving up your favourite foods. The beauty of the approach is its simplicity, which removes all the stress from eating so you can enjoy your food knowing every meal is helping you move closer to your health and happiness goal!

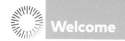

Your happiness journal explained

Here's why starting your new journal will make you happier in just a few minutes a day!

Many of us keep a diary when we're young but stop when we grow up because we don't think we have the time or energy. However, when you're busy and stressed is actually the best time to keep a daily journal because it hands you back complete control of your life, and helps give you some mental space to think about your goals and ambitions, and how to make them a reality.

We think journaling is a fantastic, life-enhancing habit that can make you feel happier instantly. And that's why it's a very important part of The SHIFT56 System, alongside the fat loss exercise and eating plan you've just read about, to help you lead a fitter, healthier and happier life right now!

We explain how you can start your new journal, and set yourself the perfect eight-week health and happiness goal, on p90 – but first we've answered some of the big journaling questions you might have.

What is journaling?
Journaling is simply taking a little time each day to write down your plans and motivations, and to reflect on your day. It's a fantastic way to take control of your day-to-day life, and give yourself regular reminders that every positive action you take – no matter how small – really does add up!

What do I need to write down?
When it's time to start keeping your daily journal, turn to p99 where you'll find each day has its own page – all you need to do is fill in the spaces. It only takes a few minutes to do, but you won't believe the difference it will make to your productivity, motivation, calmness and much more besides! To get even more out of your new journal, you should first set your eight-week health and happiness goal.

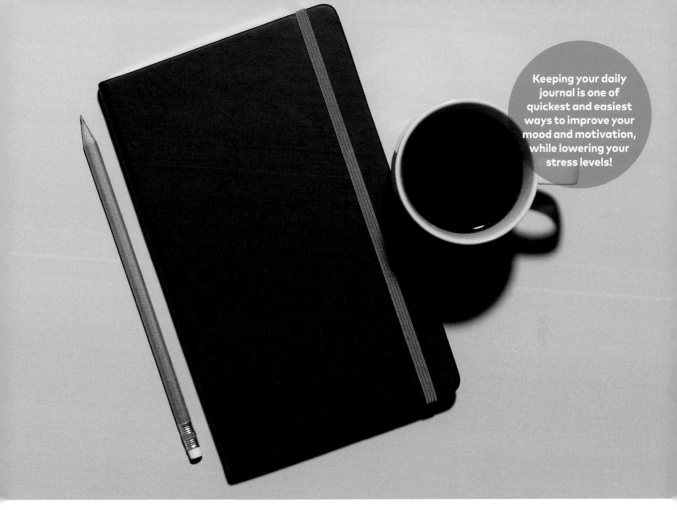

Keeping your daily journal is one of quickest and easiest ways to improve your mood and motivation, while lowering your stress levels!

Why do I need to set a goal?

Having a clearly defined, challenging yet achievable goal is one of the most important steps you can take towards living a better life. Without a goal it's impossible to make big or lasting health and happiness changes. It would be like taking a journey without a map; it doesn't matter how fast or for how long you travel, you'll probably end up going round in circles!

How do I set my goal?

Setting your overall goal, which we call your Big Picture Goal (BPG), requires you to think about what you can realistically achieve in the next eight weeks. We've explained how to choose the perfect goal for you on p100 but for now, have a think about what you want to achieve. Don't worry if it feels a little daunting or overwhelming – that's entirely normal – and remember we're here to help every step of the way!

How do I make my goal a reality?

To help you achieve your Big Picture Goal you'll set Weekly Achievable Goals, or WAGs, that break down your main goal into smaller, easier "stepping stones". Achieving your WAGs keeps you moving towards your BPG, and increases your confidence, motivation and willpower!

What tips are there to help me keep my journal?

There's lots of great tips and advice to help you get going – and keep going – with your daily journal from p94. We promise it's the simplest and easiest thing you can do today to make instant improvements to your life!

 Quick tip

Setting a realistic goal and keeping a journal are proven methods of improving your mood and mental well-being, and they'll work hand in hand with your new exercise and eating plan to help you lose body fat and make big improvements to your life. As you'll soon find out, setting weekly targets in your journal, then tracking all your positive daily actions, is the very best way to fast-track your results.

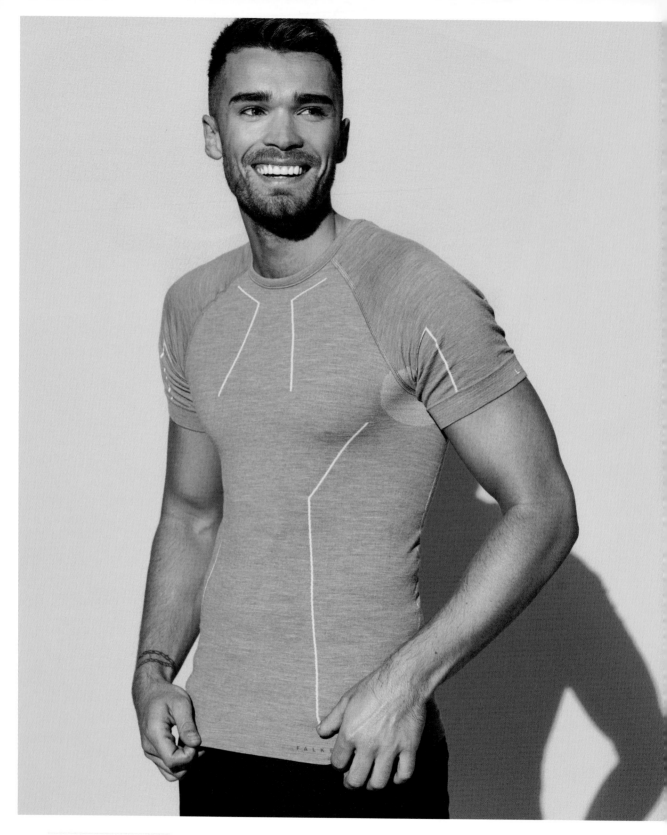

Your healthier and happier life starts now!

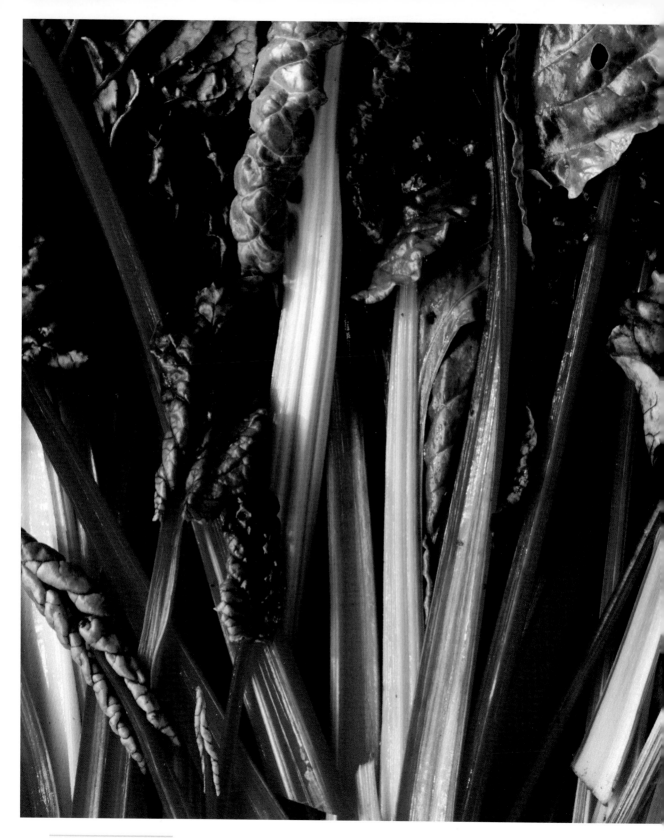

Eat smart

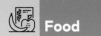

Eat smart to lose fat!

Lose weight and live happier with our smart, simple and sustainable approach to food, eating and nutrition

Food is a huge part of The SHIFT56 System, and with very good reason! Eating is something we all have to do, and gaining a better understanding of the huge impact the food you eat – and how you eat it – has on your health and happiness will empower you to start making better nutrition decisions to help you look and feel better than ever.

In this chapter you'll discover why "detox diets" actually make you fatter and sadder; why counting calories is a waste of your time (and why you need never do it again); the smarter way to eat for better health and happiness (without giving up the foods you love!); how to be more present at mealtimes (and why doing so will help you shift fat faster); the simple mind-tricks to help you stop overeating for good... and much, much more, so you can start eating for a healthy and happier life today!

Chapter Contents

Ditch the detox diet!

Want to lose fat fast? Here's why "quick-fix" diets are the worst thing you can do!

We all know the feeling: waking up the morning after the night before. Or the morning after the weekend before! Perhaps you drank too much, ate too much, or had too much of something that disagrees with you. For many people, it's at this moment – or when they face the mirror, or get on the bathroom scale, or struggle to buckle their belt – that they start thinking about a diet.

Most people want quick results: you feel bad now and want to feel better asap. But while quick-fix diets – whether they're called a "detox", a "cleanse", a "metabolic reset" or any other attention-grabbing name – promise instant results, they never work for long. Even worse, they'll make you fatter and unhappier in the long run.

How do I lose – or gain – weight?
Before we get to why quick-fix diets are so dangerous it's important to understand how we gain and lose weight. In theory, weight loss is simple. It's based on the Energy Balance Equation (we'll explain it in more detail shortly), which says that to lose weight you must consume less energy – in other words, fewer calories from food – than you burn.

We expend energy through simply being alive (our bodies burn calories at rest to keep us alive, at what's known as the basal metabolic rate or BMR), and also through everyday activities, exercise and excretion. Over time if we eat fewer calories than we burn, we lose weight; if we eat more calories than we burn, we gain weight.

This concept is important to understand because it's how all diets work. It doesn't matter if you're only eating "superfoods", having one meal a day or ten, or eat standing on your head (don't do that) – you'll lose weight only if you consume less energy than you expend. But that doesn't mean all diets are equal in helping you lose weight, or improving your health and happiness! Keep reading to discover why "detox diets" are so bad for both your body and your brain.

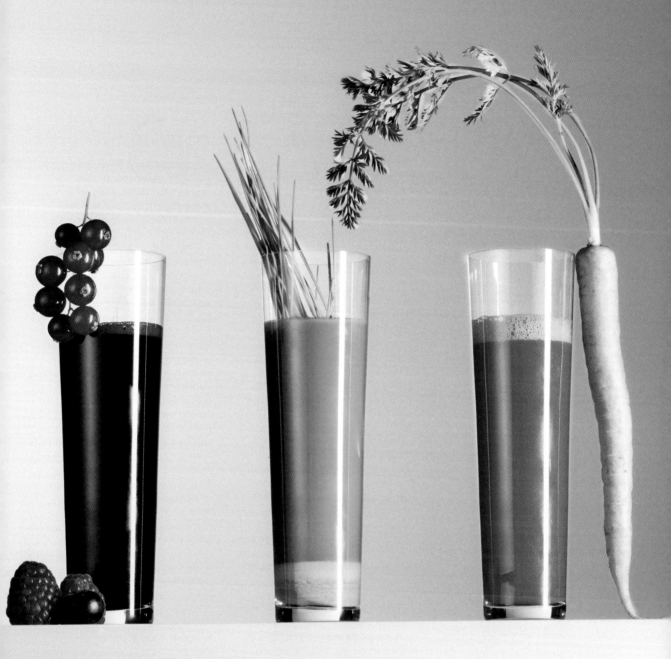

5 reasons detox diets are so dangerous

Here's why quick-fix diets will damage your health and make you fatter!

PROBLEM 1

You mess up your fluid balance

Why is this bad? Many quick-fix or fad diets "work" because when you first start restricting your food intake or cut out certain nutrients to reduce your daily calorie consumption, you will lose weight. A big problem is that it's not fat that you've lost – it's water. And that's the last thing you want to happen.

This is one reason detox diets are so incredibly dangerous. They can negatively affect your body's fluid and salt (better known as electrolyte) balance, which means you can lose a lot of water and salts very quickly. Disrupting fluid and electrolyte balance will result in dehydration, which will make you look, feel and perform far worse than normal.

Take things too far and these dangers become much more serious because your body depends on fluid and electrolyte balance for maintaining the rhythm of your heart, as well as many other very important functions.

So if you're ever tempted to try one of those so-called "detox diets", remember that you might see a lower number on the bathroom scale after a few days but any weight lost is probably water, rather than that body fat you really want to shift. And remember it's likely to make you feel tired, dehydrated and miserable – and that's about as far from living a healthier and happier life as you can be.

PROBLEM 2

You starve your body of nutrients

Why is this bad? Almost all quick-fix diets are based on severely restricting your daily calorie intake by cutting out specific types of foods or eliminating food groups entirely.

This means that these diets don't provide some, or even many, of the essential nutrients your body needs to function at its best – whether that's fats, protein or vitamins and minerals. So they will dramatically affect how "healthy" you look and feel.

You may suffer physical signs, such as dry, pale or dull skin, aching joints and muscles, feelings of lethargy and weakness, or trouble falling and staying asleep, as well as a wide range of mental symptoms, not limited to constant hunger, low energy and constant fatigue, bad moods, and dire levels of focus, motivation and concentration.

All you will think about is food and your next meal, not to mention that pit-of-your-stomach disappointment about what that next meal is going to be!

This will make you feel absolutely awful in the short term and cause you to question whether all these negative side effects are worth it. (They're not.) But it has an even more serious impact on your long-term health, fitness and general well-being.

PROBLEM 3

Your metabolism slows down

Why is this bad? Your body's job, evolutionarily speaking, is to stop you starving to death – a very real risk until relatively recently. So your body pays very close attention to how much you're eating.

When you suddenly start eating less your body makes adjustments to prevent starvation. Your metabolism slows down to conserve energy, and many other changes occur. Your digestive tract moves food through more slowly to extract as much energy and as many nutrients as possible (which can cause digestive issues, such as bloating or constipation); your repair and recovery processes slow down so you don't heal as fast; and there's a reduced production of important hormones, including the primary sex hormones oestrogen, progesterone and testosterone.

When your metabolism slows, your body decides you need even less energy to survive, which means you now must further reduce your calorie intake from food to get into that calorie deficit to lose weight! This creates a vicious cycle in which your body, over time, requires fewer and fewer calories to function, making it harder to lose weight even when you're eating far less than before. This is really bad for your weight loss ambition. Why? Keep reading.

PROBLEM 4

Your appetite roars back

Why is this bad? Have you ever wondered what makes you feel hungry? Or full? Appetite is controlled by a series of feedback loops in the digestive system and the brain. There are also sensors in our fat cells that tell our brain how full our fat stores are. If there's a lack of food being eaten, these feedback loops and sensors compensate by making you really hungry. The "if you're standing between me and the fridge I can't be held responsible for my actions" kind of hungry!

No matter how strong your willpower and motivation, your brain's "don't starve" system is always stronger.

Eventually you quit the diet (because it's unsustainable and you're miserable) and resume eating normally. But you now need fewer calories than before because of your slower metabolism, so you gain back the weight you lost – and more – because your brain is sending all the excess energy to fill up your fat stores in an effort to make sure you don't "starve" again. You'll think about food more often – and hence eat more too. This is a major reason so many people end up yo-yo dieting and gain body fat rather than losing it.

PROBLEM 5

You get stuck in a vicious cycle

Why is this bad? There are many physiological problems caused by quick-fix diets, but one of the biggest is the damaging habits that they cause people to adopt.

To lose weight and keep it off, you must make some simple and sustainable habit changes. We'll get to how you can do that really easily soon, but first here are some of the worst habits that are forged by quick-fix diets.

- You learn to either be "on" a diet or "off" it – there is nothing in between

- You only ever experience a very short period of weight loss "success", if any

- You experience long periods of "failure", and feelings of guilt or frustration that add to your unhappiness

- You start to develop a damaging relationship with food and think obsessively about eating

- You forget how to "trust" your body to know how it's really feeling, and don't trust yourself to make smart food choices

- You end up in one of two equally bad scenarios: either living a life adhering to a very strict set of eating rules, or suffering from a complete loss of control over your diet and your life

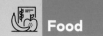
The calorie question

Here's how many calories you need to eat each day to achieve your health goal

If you've heard it once, you've heard it a thousand times: losing weight is all about calories in versus calories out. It's pretty simple: eat fewer calories than you burn and you lose weight; eat more calories than you burn and you gain weight. It's called the Energy Balance Equation and here it is:

Change in body stores = Energy In – Energy Out

The equation says "body stores" rather than "bodyweight" because body stores refers to the bodily tissues, such as muscle and fat, that are affected by a positive or negative energy balance equation. "Bodyweight" can be significantly impacted by changes in body water – but those changes are temporary.

Estimating your energy needs

Determining your daily energy requirements can be very complex, requiring you to input your height, weight, age, sex, activity levels, goals and other data into mathematical equations.

But there's an easier way: use this chart! It gets you incredibly close to the same total daily calorie number with a fraction of the time and effort! The formula is in pounds (lb) – there are 14lb in one stone. In general women should use the smaller multipliers in each box and men the larger one. If you know your weight in kilos, multiply it by 2.2 to convert it to pounds.

Your activity level	YOUR GOAL Lose Fat	Maintain Weight	Gain Muscle
Lightly Active (<3 hrs/wk)	Bodyweight (lb) x 10-12	Bodyweight (lb) x 12-14	Bodyweight (lb) x 16-18
Moderately Active (3-6 hrs/wk)	Bodyweight (lb) x 12-14	Bodyweight (lb) x 14-16	Bodyweight (lb) x 18-20
Very Active (>6 hrs/wk)	Bodyweight (lb) x 14-16	Bodyweight (lb) x 16-18	Bodyweight (lb) x 20-22

Putting theory into practice

To understand how this works in real life, here are a couple of examples.

EXAMPLE 1

A 160lb (11st 6lb), moderately active woman wanting to lose fat

She would estimate her calorie needs by multiplying her weight in pounds x 12, which is 160 x 12 = 1,920.

To lose weight she would require approximately 1,920 calories daily.

EXAMPLE 2

A 190lb (13st 8lb), moderately active man wanting to gain muscle

He would estimate his calorie needs by multiplying his weight in pounds x 20, which is 190 x 20 = 3,800.

To gain weight he would require approximately 3,800 calories daily.

Simple, right? Yes – except these calorie targets are only very rough starting points. And an even bigger problem is that accurately estimating the calories you've actually eaten, and those you've burned, is far more complicated and difficult than you've been led to believe.

Quick tip Determining your daily calorie needs based on your weight, goal, activity level and gender is easy, but by itself it's not actionable. All you get is a number, which may not be accurate because accurately estimating how many calories you eat and burn each day is almost impossible, and we'll explain why on the next page. This is why a nutrition plan based on calorie counting is a flawed approach, but that's OK because we have a far better and easier approach to eating that'll make you look and feel fantastic!

Why calorie counts don't add up!

Here's why estimating your daily calorie intake can lead you on a wild goose chase

You now know a simple way to estimate your approximate daily calorie need. You also know that to lose or gain weight you must be in a daily calorie deficit or surplus. So the best approach to build the body you want is to count the calories you eat and the ones you burn, right? Not so fast. While counting calories is a very popular weight loss strategy, it isn't as effective as you may think. Let's go back to the Energy Balance Equation, which as you know looks like this: Change in body stores = Energy In – Energy Out. When we look more closely at this equation, some pretty big problems begin to emerge.

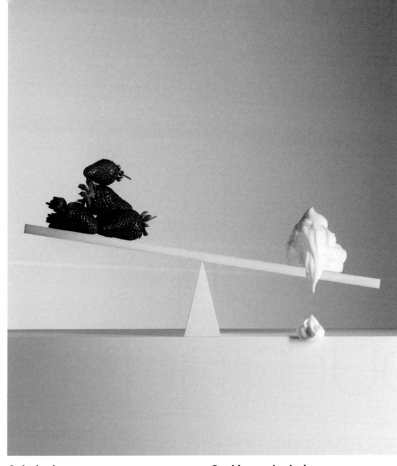

Calories in

First, for the "Energy In" part of the equation, you must figure out how many calories are in the foods you want to eat, and that requires handbooks, websites, databases and maths – just to have your lunch!

Then you must assume that these calorie data sources are correct. They're often not: research shows they can be out by 20% or more because of incorrect labelling, laboratory measurement error or food quality.

The amount of processing a food has undergone is another key factor in your energy intake. You'll absorb fewer calories from minimally processed foods such as fruits, vegetables, lean meats, nuts and whole grains than from highly processed foods, such as oils, sugar, refined grains and pre-packaged foods. Surprised? Wait, there's more.

Cooking and calories

How you prepare and cook food also affects the total number of calories your body absorbs. You absorb about 47 calories from a raw egg, 196 calories from 4oz of raw steak, and 101 calories from a medium raw potato (not that we'd recommend eating them!). Cook those foods and you'll absorb around 74 calories from the egg, 240 calories from the steak and 193 calories from the potato. Of course, these actual numbers vary significantly depending on when, where and how the food was grown, shipped and stored, as well as cooking method, time and many other factors!

Finally, we have trillions of bacteria in our guts that affect our body in hundreds of ways, and research suggests that people with higher proportions of certain bacteria can absorb up to 150 more calories per day than people with a lower proportion.

Refining the formula

What does this all mean? That the "Energy In" part of the equation actually looks like this:

**Energy In =
Actual Calories Eaten –
Calories Not Absorbed**

Therefore, the "Energy In" side is very hard – if not impossible – to calculate accurately. It can be wrong by as much as 20%, a potentially huge margin of error in something so important to your chances of successfully achieving the body you want.

Quick tip

Calorie counts and nutrition labels are imprecise, and the amount of processing a food undergoes affects how many calories you absorb. How, when and where our food is grown, shipped, stored, prepped and cooked can all affect its calorie load, and people vary in the number of calories they absorb from the food they eat. Ultimately, estimating your calorie intake is a flawed approach and, as you are about to find out on the next page, so is estimating your calorie expenditure!

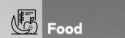
How many calories are you burning?

Here's why accurately calculating your energy expenditure is as difficult as guessing your intake

You now know how to estimate your daily calorie needs, but also the many problems of calculating the number of calories you actually eat each day.

Now we're going to look at the "Energy Out" part of the Energy Balance Equation, because there are some big issues with that too (don't worry – we'll get to the solution to this calorie conundrum soon!). First things first: there are four ways your body burns calories, as you'll see on the next page...

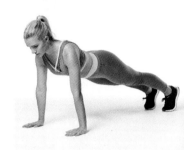

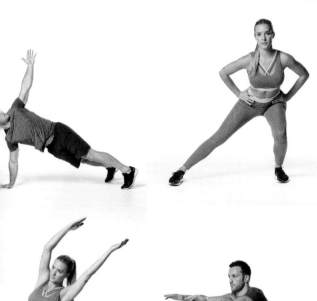
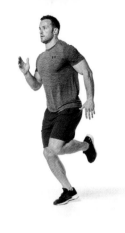

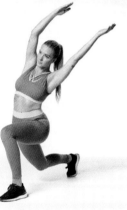
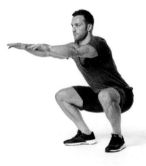
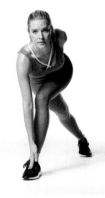
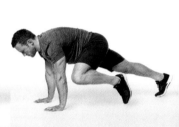

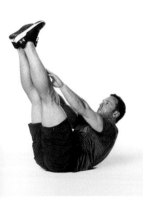
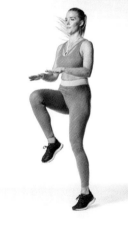
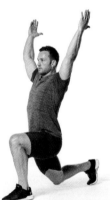
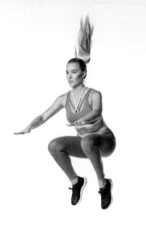

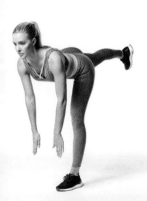
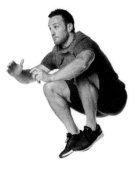
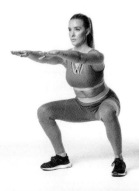
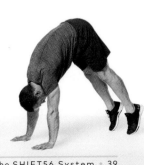

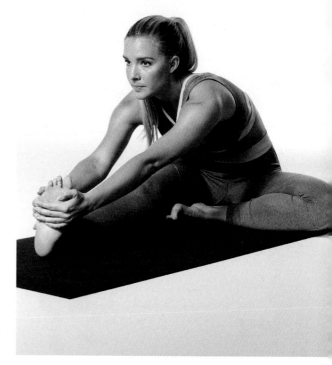

1 Resting metabolic rate (RMR)

RMR is the number of calories you burn each day at rest, just breathing, thinking and living. It represents around 60% of your daily energy expenditure and depends on your weight, body composition, sex, age, genetic predisposition, and the bacteria in your gut. In general a bigger body has a higher RMR, yet it can vary up to 15% from person to person. If you weigh 200lb (14st 4lb) with an RMR of 1,905 calories, someone else who weighs exactly the same as you could burn 286 more (or fewer) calories each day with no more (or less) effort!

2 Thermic effect of eating (TEE)

That's right, it takes energy to process food. TEE is the number of calories you burn by eating, digesting and absorbing food and it represents around 5-10% of your daily energy expenditure. You'll burn more calories digesting and absorbing protein (around 20-30% of its calories) than carbs (5-6%) or fats (3%), and you also burn more calories digesting natural whole foods than you do highly processed foods. If you've ever had the "meat sweats" or felt hot after a big protein-rich meal, that's TEE in action!

3 Physical activity (PA)

PA is the calories you burn from purposeful exercise, such as walking, running, going to the gym, gardening, cycling or other physical activities. Obviously, how much energy you expend through PA is determined by how much you intentionally move around.

4 Non-exercise activity thermogenesis (NEAT)

NEAT is the calories you burn through fidgeting, staying upright and all other physical movements that don't count as PA. NEAT output can vary tremendously between individuals. In studies where people are overfed, some individuals burn off 70% of those extra calories through NEAT alone, while others actually burn less! And in studies where people are underfed, some subjects' NEAT output dropped dramatically (making it harder for them to lose weight), while others had minimal change in their NEAT output (making it easier for them to lose weight). Ultimately, NEAT output can vary by as many as 2,000 calories between individuals!

Changing the equation

All this means the "Energy Out" side of the Energy Balance Equation should actually look more like this:

> Energy Out = Resting Metabolic Rate (RMR)
>   + Thermic Effect of Eating (TEE)
>   + Physical Activity (PA)
>   + Non-Exercise Activity Thermogenesis (NEAT)

Each of these four factors is highly variable and constantly changing, making the "Energy Out" side of the Energy Balance Equation as hard to calculate as the "Energy In" side.

So, while the equation seems simple in theory, all these variables make it very hard – perhaps impossible – to know or control exactly how much energy you're taking in, absorbing, burning and storing each day.

Here's what the Energy Balance Equation actually looks like:

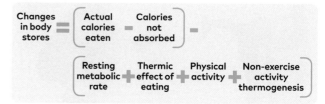

Mission impossible!

Even if all the variables in the Energy Balance Equation were static, it is still very complicated to comprehend. But these variables are never static, not least because when one variable changes it will cause a change in others.

This is a good thing, of course. The human metabolism evolved to keep us alive when food was scarce. But this means that – as we saw on p30 – when "Energy In" goes down, "Energy Out" goes down too. In other words, your metabolism slows in response to eating less, so you burn fewer calories. This doesn't happen in everybody, nor in a uniform way, but it's how the metabolic system is supposed to work.

To illustrate this point, here's how your body adjusts the Energy Balance Equation to prevent rapid weight loss in response to a dramatic reduction in your calorie intake, such as when going on a "quick-fix" or "detox" diet.

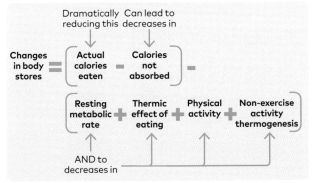

Tracking your energy expenditure

Ultimately, estimating your calorie expenditure is fraught with uncertainties and potential errors. As we've discussed, the food you eat affects how many calories you burn (digesting protein causes more calories to be burned than carbs or fats), and unprocessed whole foods provide fewer dietary calories and require more calories to digest than highly processed foods.

But there's more. A single night of sleep deprivation can cause your metabolism to burn as much as 20% fewer calories the following day. Just to complicate matters, your brain will seek out high-sugar and high-fat foods in response to tiredness!

Your previous weight history also influences how many calories you burn. If you've ever been overweight or obese, your metabolic rate may be about 10% lower than someone of the same weight, age, sex and body composition who was never overweight or obese.

So it's almost impossible to accurately know how many calories you burn each day. Even fitness trackers, which are excellent at monitoring your heart rate, have been found to miscalculate calorie expenditure by up to 30%!

Just like your "Energy In" number, your "Energy Out" estimate can also be wrong by as much as 20% – a massive margin of error for something so important to your health and happiness!

Quick tip

Calorie expenditure estimates are imprecise and people burn calories at unique and variable rates. Metabolic responses to overeating and undereating vary tremendously between individuals, and other factors including your previous weight history also affect how many calories you burn daily. This means that calorie counting is a fundamentally flawed approach. Luckily there is a better way. Turn the page to find out more!

Flexible Eating: eat smarter for life!

Taking a flexible approach to food is the best way to eat for health and happiness

Scientific researchers and nutrition experts have spent decades trying to understand the best ways to help people lose weight and then, crucially, keep it off. Two of The SHIFT56 System's contributing editors, Brian St Pierre and Krista Scott-Dixon, work for Precision Nutrition, the world's leading nutritional education company.

PN has worked with more than 100,000 people to help them to lose weight and improve their health and performance, so PN's experts have a wealth of knowledge about what works and what doesn't, and why people succeed or fail in their attempt to become leaner, fitter and healthier. So what's PN's secret? Consistency! Turn the page to find out more.

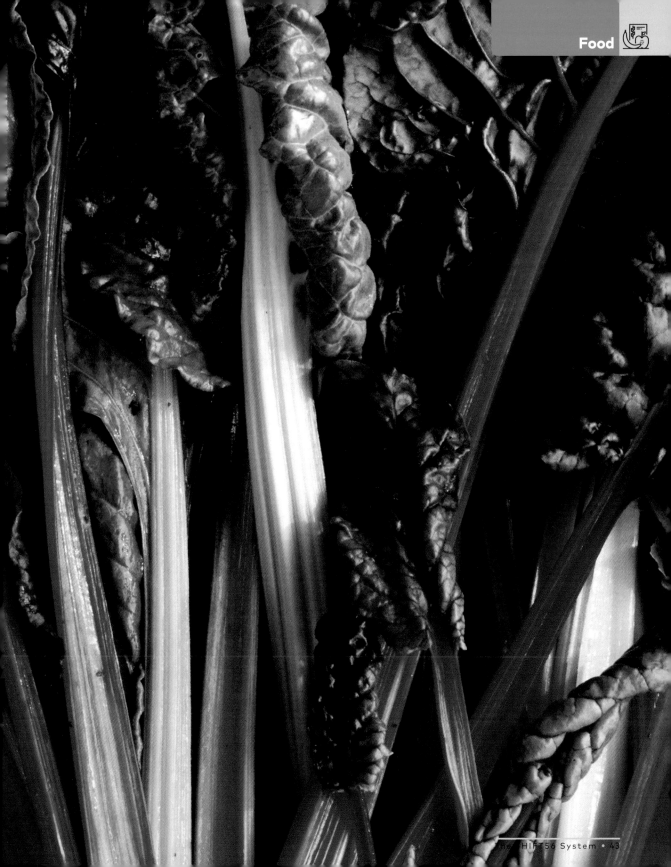

Consistency is everything

Consistency might not sound sexy, but in both research and real life it's what ultimately helps people control their calorie intake and manage hunger comfortably.

By "comfortably" we mean causing the least amount of tension between your body composition goals (your health and fitness) and the lifestyle you desire (your happiness).

What never works is having two competing desires, like the guy who wants to have a six-pack but still drink four pints every night, or the woman who wants to drop from size 16 to 12 but still eat takeaways four nights a week. In these examples those two desires actively compete against one another, and that's what creates frustration and unhappiness because you're pursuing an impossible outcome.

Finding a nutrition plan that allows you to live your preferred lifestyle *and* achieve your health goals is critical to achieving long-lasting happiness. And we call that plan Flexible Eating.

Perfection is impossible!

Our Flexible Eating plan means you don't need to eat "perfectly" 100% of the time to succeed. In fact, most people do best in both the short term and the long term when eating well 80-90% of the time: 80% works for more modest goals; and 90% for achieving more challenging goals.

Remember, the "all or nothing" approach rarely gets you all – it usually gets you nothing!

The Flexible Eating approach removes the pressure of trying to be "perfect" all day, every day (which is impossible anyway!). And, crucially, it allows you to eat for pure and simple pleasure 10-20% of the time – that's one of the best things about our eating plan.

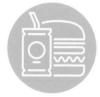

There are no "bad foods"

Allowing yourself to eat for pleasure means foods are no longer categorised as either "good" or "bad". Such a black-and-white approach "moralises" foods and makes you think about certain foods in terms of guilt and regret instead of contentment and joy. That's no way to live your life if you're seeking greater health and happiness (you can read more on guilt-free eating on p66).

Instead of "good" or "bad" foods, think instead of foods falling on a spectrum of "eat more often" and "eat less often". Minimally processed foods such as lean protein, vegetables, fruits, whole grains and healthy fats are foods to eat more often. However, as we mentioned, this doesn't mean "eat always".

Highly processed foods and drinks such as chips, crisps, biscuits, cakes, pizza, bacon, ice cream, chocolate, fizzy drinks and alcohol should be consumed less often. But, again, this doesn't mean "never".

Thinking about food in these terms, and then using our Perfect Portion meal-building approach (which is explained in full on p50), makes it incredibly easy to choose "eat more often" foods, while also making those "eat less often" foods a more enjoyable and guilt-free experience when you do consume them. And who doesn't want that?

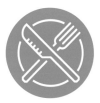

Flexibility for life

One big advantage of Flexible Eating is that if you're going to a wedding, party, work conference or other event where the food is likely to be in the "eat less often" category, it's not a problem! Use it as an opportunity to enjoy, in reasonable amounts, some of those foods that are good for the soul. You'll enjoy these foods guilt-free, have a fun and relaxing social experience – and still be moving towards your health and happiness goals!

Of course, if you don't approach Flexible Eating with purpose and awareness, then it can become a slippery slope on which you find it easy to rationalise a greater inclusion of "eat less often" foods at the expense of "eat more often" foods. You need to be honest with yourself, and recognise that long-term consistency is what really matters. If you get this right, you can follow this approach and get great results – without ever having to "diet" again!

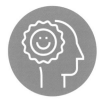

Go easy on yourself!

Before we explain our Perfect Portion meal strategy that will help you eat for a healthier and happier life, it's important to realise that your Flexible Eating approach needs to be adapted based on your current goals and life circumstances.

For instance, if you've recently had a child, or are spending more time looking after elderly or ill relatives, there's a strong case for being a bit more relaxed about hitting that 80% consistency target and perhaps "dialling it down" for a while.

But maybe your kids have just started school or left home, or you've found yourself newly single. This could be a good time to increase your consistency a little – maybe "dialling it up" closer to 90% consistency than 80% – to push yourself a bit harder and get even better results.

This concept of "dialling" up or down your consistency based on your current circumstances is really beneficial because it helps you stay on the right track for the majority of the time, and reminds you that you don't have to completely throw in the towel when life suddenly goes crazy! All you have to do is dial it down until you have the time and energy to dial it back up again.

Quick tip

The "all or nothing" mentality never gets us all; it gets us nothing. So start at that 80% consistency level, then dial up or dial down to fit your current goals and life circumstances. Be self-compassionate and not self-critical, and that consistency level will deliver success in a sane, sustainable and enjoyable manner. Next we're going to look at what actually makes up the food you eat, and then we'll explain our Perfect Portion system. This is the meal-building approach that will help you eat for a healthier and happier life – in the easiest way possible!

What's in your food?

Here's a guide to the major and minor components in the food you eat – and why they're so important

Every single thing we eat is a combination of different compounds. Most natural, unprocessed food consists primarily of water: a banana is 75% water, a potato is 79% water and a chicken breast, which most people think of as pure protein, can be up to 75% water. But this isn't actually that surprising when you consider you are around 70% water – so you're more H_2O than anything else!

After water the next most common compound in natural foods will be a macronutrient – there are three of them – or a combination of macronutrients along with certain micronutrients. Turn the page to find out more.

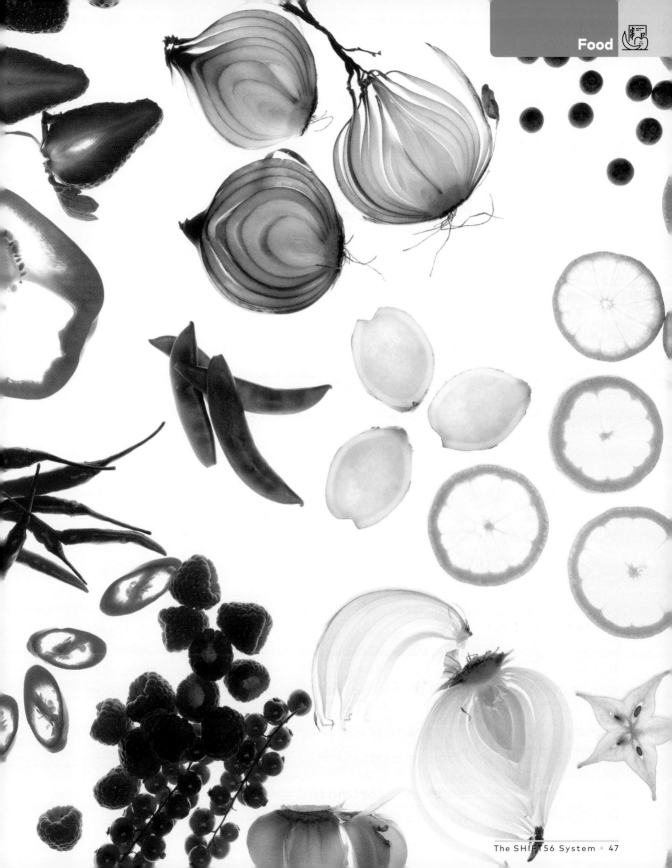

What are macronutrients?

Macronutrients are the three main groups of chemical compounds that make up the food we eat. They are protein, fats and carbohydrates.

What are micronutrients?

Micronutrients are chemical compounds such as vitamins, minerals and phytonutrients (plant-based nutrients) in food. They are found in much smaller quantities than macronutrients, and we only need them in very small amounts.

MACRONUTRIENTS

Protein

After water, most of what makes you, well, *you* is made from proteins, and all proteins are made from amino acids. There are many types of amino acid, most of which your body can manufacture itself when required, but there are nine amino acids your body can't synthesise. They're called "essential amino acids" and you must get them from food. Most foods contain at least small (or "trace") amounts of protein, but these are some of the most protein-rich foods.

Animal sources

- poultry (chicken, turkey, duck, goose) and eggs
- red meat (beef, pork, lamb)
- wild game (venison, rabbit, pheasant)
- fish and shellfish
- dairy (milk, cheese, yogurt)

Plant sources

- beans and legumes
- tofu, tempeh and other soy products
- nuts and seeds (though these are generally much higher in fat than protein)
- some grains such as quinoa, amaranth and wild rice (though these are much higher in carbohydrates than protein)

How much do I need?

A good target is about 0.8g-1g of protein per kilogram of bodyweight per day, but you may need more if you're active, older, pregnant or breastfeeding, or ill or injured.

Carbohydrates

There are many types of carbohydrates and they're mainly found in plant-based foods. Some carbs are very simple molecules, such as sugars, which are the most basic form. Others are much more complicated and are called complex carbohydrates. Starches, which are found in potatoes and beans, are one type of complex carb, as is fibre.

The more "simple" the carbohydrate the easier it is to digest and absorb. In general, when eating for better health and fitness you want to prioritise consuming complex carbohydrates because they are slower-digesting and more nutrient-rich than simple carbs.

Our bodies can't completely break down some types of complex carbs, such as insoluble fibre or resistant starch, but the bacteria in our gut love it and make other beneficial compounds from it. Fibre and resistant starch are often known as "prebiotics": they're food sources that nourish our "good" gut bacteria. Fibre also helps move things through our intestinal tract.

Higher-fibre foods include fruits and vegetables, whole grains, beans and legumes, and nuts and seeds, and resistant starch is found in beans, green bananas, and many other plant-based foods.

Water

Make sure you're drinking enough to stay fit and focused

We are about 70% water and can't live long without it. Regulating thirst and maintaining the balance of fluids and electrolytes are two of your body's most vital tasks. We take in water through drinking, obviously, but also through eating fluid-rich fruits and veg, and we lose it through breathing, sweating and excretion.

You've probably heard you need to drink eight glasses of water per day, but there's no evidence to support that. There's also no reason to be peeing "clear" urine: a light yellow colour is fine.

There are simple ways to avoid dehydration: drink a big glass of water as soon as you wake up; pay more attention to thirst; drink more during exercise or in hot or humid conditions; choose water as your go-to drink (instead of alcohol or caffeinated drinks); and check your urine colour (the darker it is, the more dehydrated you are). If you often forget to drink enough water – you may notice you feel mentally and physically tired – fill up a water bottle at the beginning of the day, keep it close and take a big gulp every time you look at it!

Best sources of fibre and micronutrient-rich carbs

- Sweet and starchy vegetables (winter squashes, beetroot)
- Starchy tubers (potatoes, sweet potatoes, yams)
- Whole grains (rice, wheat, oats)
- Beans and legumes
- Fruit

How much do I need?
That depends on myriad factors, including your activity levels: you need more carbs if you are physically active and/or trying to build muscle. While some people do benefit from a lower-carb diet, most people look, feel and perform better from eating at least some carbs, especially the nutrient-rich, higher-fibre types.

> If you eat processed foods you will consume substances that are technically edible, such as preservatives, binders and colouring agents, but these are not really "food"

Fats
The main three types of dietary fat are saturated, monounsaturated and polyunsaturated (see below). They differ from one another by the number and frequency of the carbon atoms that bond them, but we don't need to worry about that! You just need to know that fats are an essential macronutrient and you need to consume them for optimal health (it's yet another reason why very low-fat "detox diets" make you look and feel so bad!).

How much do I need?
Most people do best with 25-35% of their total daily calories coming from a wide variety of healthy fat sources. Omega-3 fatty acids, particularly EPA and DHA, are special types of fats found in oily fish, seafood and some plant sources. They can help you lose weight, boost brain function, reduce inflammation, and improve both your physical and mental health – they're all-round performers!

You may have noticed that processed cooking oils, margarine and cooking sprays don't appear here and with good reason! Most "long life" cooking oils and margarines are heavily processed and contain types of fat called "trans fats" that aren't found in nature, so your body doesn't know how to process them. Research increasingly suggests trans fats contribute to many health problems.

MICRONUTRIENTS
Vitamins and minerals come in many forms and what we think of as a "vitamin" or a "mineral" is actually a group of molecules that are chemically similar, but sufficiently different to do different jobs in the body. For example "vitamin A" is actually a family of molecules, and the carotenoid forms of vitamin A (such as beta-carotene) are water-soluble, found mainly in plants (such as carrots), and not very well absorbed; while the retinoid forms of vitamin A are fat-soluble, found mostly in animal foods (such as egg yolks) and are well absorbed.

We absorb minerals such as calcium, iron and magnesium from dairy and meat better than from leafy greens, which come in harder-to-digest forms. This is one reason why it's important to eat a wide variety of foods: each food has a unique chemical "fingerprint" of micronutrients that contributes to our good health.

You may think taking a multi-vitamin or multi-mineral supplement helps you avoid deficiencies, but taking more vitamin and/or mineral pills is not usually better or healthier. Instead, focus on improving the quality and variety of your food choices so that you get your vitamins and minerals in the form that nature intended.

The 3 types of fat

Most fat sources contain more than one type of dietary fat, but these foods are particularly high in one type

Saturated fats
- Butter and high-fat dairy (eg cheese)
- Most animal fats
- Coconut and coconut oil
- Egg yolk
- Cacao butter

Monounsaturated fats
- Avocado
- Olives and olive oil
- Peanuts
- Many types of nuts, such as pecans and almonds

Polyunsaturated fats
- Many types of seeds such as flax, chia, sesame and sunflower seeds
- Oily fish such as salmon, herring, and mackerel

The Perfect Portion plan!

Here's how to start eating for greater health and happiness without counting calories!

So we've established that the whole concept of "calorie counting" is fundamentally flawed, with a potentially huge margin of error on both the "Energy In" and "Energy Out" sides of the equation.

And you now know that our Flexible Eating strategy – where you eat well around 80-90% of the time and for pure pleasure 10-20% of the time – is the smart, sensible and sustainable eating approach for better health and happiness!

Ultimately calories do matter – because to lose weight you need to be in a "calorie deficit" so your body starts tapping into fat stores for fuel – but counting calories doesn't work, and is also a real drag! Who wants to be digging out measuring cups whenever they're hungry? Or be constantly cleaning food scales? Or spending good money on apps and online services to track those less-than-accurate calorie numbers? No wonder so many people quit calorie counting almost as soon as they start!

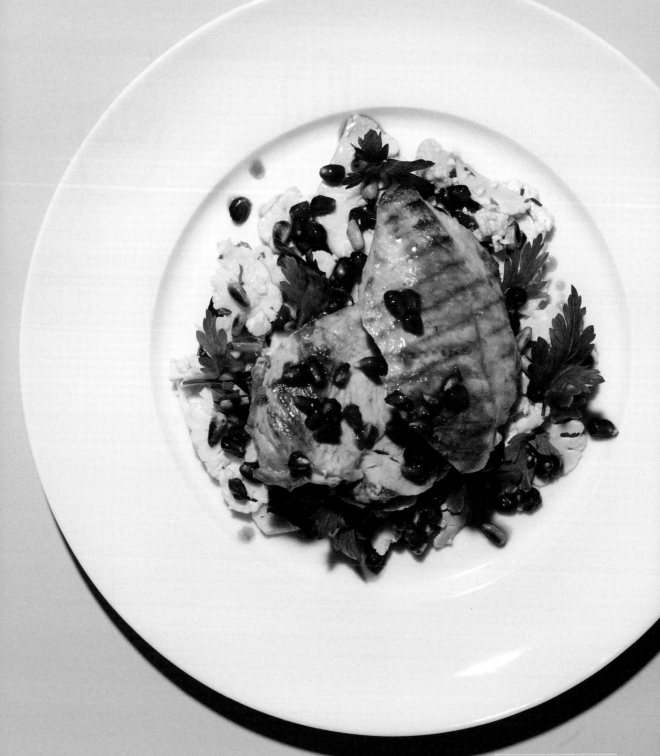

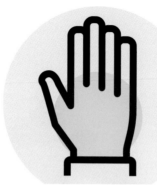

Your palm determines your protein portions

Your palm provides 20-30g of protein

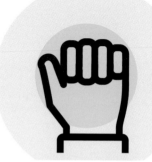

Your fist determines your veggie portions

Your fist provides about 1 cup of vegetables (weight varies depending on the veg!)

The Perfect Portion approach

Fortunately, you need never count calories again because there is a better and easier way to know which foods you should be eating and how much of them. It's called the Perfect Portion approach, and all you need is your own hand and the ability to count to two!

The Perfect Portion approach empowers you to know exactly which food groups should make up each of your meals, and in exactly the right amounts you need. Here's what you need to know.

Why it works

It might seem strange at first, but using your hands to work out your perfect portion sizes makes perfect sense! First, your hands are convenient: they're by your side at work lunches, restaurants, social occasions – wherever you go, they go! Second, hands are scaled to the individual. Bigger people need more food, and tend to have bigger hands, so they get larger portions. Smaller people need less food, and tend to have smaller hands, so they get smaller portions. Third, it helps you meet your specific protein, vegetable, carb, fat and energy needs at each meal without having to count a single calorie or weigh a single gram of food!

How it works

If you're moderately active, here's a great way to start using the Perfect Portion approach. A moderately active man needs a total daily intake of...

- 6-8 palms of protein-dense foods
- 6-8 fists of vegetables
- 6-8 cupped handfuls of carb-dense foods
- 6-8 thumbs of fat-dense foods

A moderately active woman needs a total daily intake of...

- 4-6 palms of protein-dense foods
- 4-6 fists of vegetables
- 4-6 cupped handfuls of carb-dense foods
- 4-6 thumbs of fat-dense foods

This makes it very easy to appropriately portion each meal. For instance, if you eat three or four meals a day, the starting point for putting together each meal would be as follows...

Men
- 2 palms of protein-dense foods
- 2 fists of vegetables
- 2 cupped handfuls of carb-dense foods
- 2 thumbs of fat-dense foods.

Women
- 1 palm of protein-dense foods
- 1 fist of vegetables
- 1 cupped handful of carb-dense foods
- 1 thumb of fat-dense foods

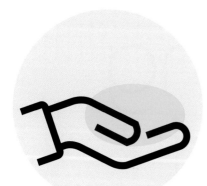

Your cupped hand determines your carb portions

Your cupped hand provides 20-30g of carbs

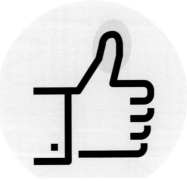

Your thumb determine your fat portions

Your thumb provides 7-12g of fat

Why do we love the Perfect Portion approach to eating so much? The reason is simple: it enables you to control your daily calorie intake almost as accurately as calorie counting, but without all the hassle and stress of kitchen scales, apps, calculators, notebooks and handbooks.

It also empowers you to be much more flexible about what you decide to eat because you can easily substitute one type of protein, carbs, fats or vegetables for another, without giving a second thought to calories!

So, you fancy a palm of steak instead of a palm of chicken or tuna or turkey? Cool! Go for it. You want a fist of carrots instead of a fist of broccoli, cauliflower or green beans? You got it! No problem. You'd prefer a cupped handful of roast potatoes instead of cupped handful of rice? Do it! Have want you want!

It really is that simple. Every single meal you eat will be determined by what you fancy or what you're craving. Not only can you say goodbye to calorie counting, you can also wave goodbye to rigid and restrictive meal plans that dictate exactly what you have to eat and when you have to eat it.

That's not a sustainable approach. This is. Which is why eating for a healthier and happier body has never been so easy!

Quick tip

Using your hands to choose appropriate portion sizes for each meal is incredibly easy and stress-free because your hands are (a) always with you and (b) scaled to your size, and so they do the macronutrient and calorie maths for you! This approach also allows for simple adjustments to personalise the Perfect Portion approach to make it even more perfect for your current health and fitness goals – and we'll get to that on the next page!

Personalising the Perfect Portion plan

Achieve your health goals faster with some simple tweaks to our better-eating guide!

The Perfect Portion approach to meals is a fantastic way to eat for better health and happiness because it does away with counting calories and categorising foods as either good or bad!

But that's not all it does. Another big advantage of this approach is that it allows you to make adjustments to your portions easily to make them even more perfect for your goals. Turn the page to find out how to do this and start benefitting from the Perfect Portion plan.

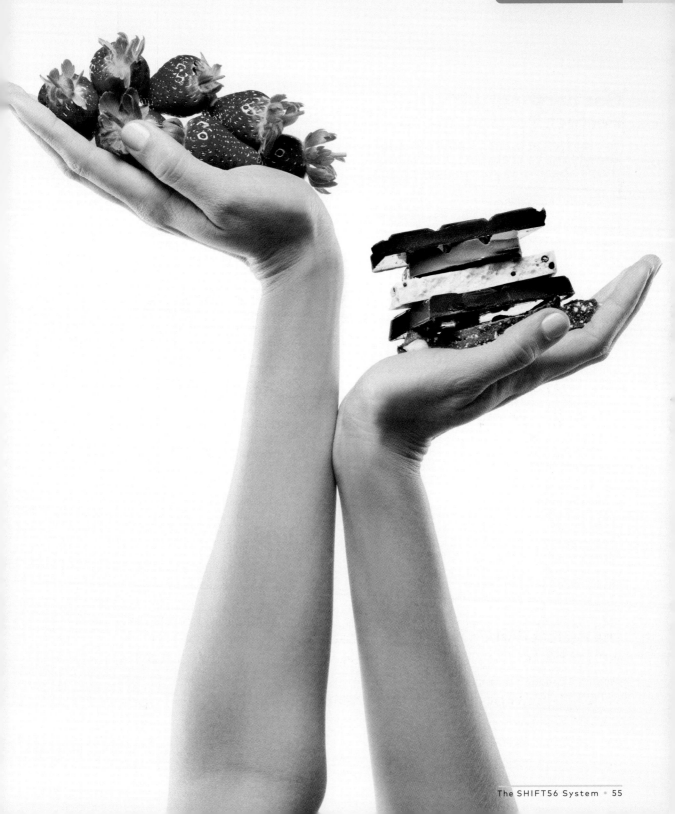

Get personal with the Perfect Portion approach

You know the basics – now use that knowledge to create a smart plan that's specific to you and your goals

It's important to remember that our portion recommendations are starting points to help you easily meet your protein, vegetable, carb, fat and energy needs without any stress or pressure – and that adjusting your portions couldn't be easier. Here's how you can do just that based on your goals.

- Women who want to lose body fat or who are lightly active might need to remove 1-3 cupped handfuls of carbs and/or 1-3 thumbs of fats from their daily intake

- Men who want to lose body fat or who are lightly active might need to remove 2-4 cupped handfuls of carbs and/or 2-4 thumbs of fats from their daily intake

- Women who want to gain lean mass or who are very active might need to add 1-4 cupped handfuls of carbs and/or 1-4 thumbs of fats to their daily intake

- Men who want to gain lean mass or who are very active might need to add 2-6 cupped handfuls of carbs and/or 2-6 thumbs of fats to their daily intake

Getting personal!
With these adjustments we have moved beyond starting points to a plan that's more tailored towards specific goals and activity levels. However, you can still adjust your portion sizes based on hunger, fullness, goals, overall activity level and, most importantly, results. What does that mean? It's really simple: you adjust your portions based on the results you are actually getting!

So, if you're not losing fat fast enough (around ½-1% of your bodyweight a week is a realistic target), remove more carb and/or fat portions. Or if you're not gaining muscle quickly enough (around ¾-1.5% bodyweight a month is a realistic target), add more carb and/or fat portions. Reassess your results and progress every couple of weeks – and keep making those tweaks!

Example Menus
Here's how your personalised portion approach might look on your plate

Knowing you should eat a palm of protein and a fist of vegetables with every meal is great, but what does this actually look like on a meal-by-meal basis? To give a clearer indication, we've created six example daily menus based on different health goals.

We've even provided some estimated nutrition facts for those of you who just have to know the calories and macronutrient count, although we can't stress enough that you should not worry about these numbers! This is simply to show that using our hand-sized portion guidelines has taken care of them for you.

Remember these are just examples. As you now know, your actual portion sizes will depend on the size of your hand, your hunger and fullness cues, your activity level and goals and, crucially, your results.

You'll notice that the fat loss menus have a cupped handful of carbs and/or a thumb of fats removed from some meals, and the muscle-gain menus have a cupped handful of carbs and/or a thumb of fats added to some meals. Again, these are just examples and you may have to adjust them to get the results you want.

Meal Plan 1

For a **woman** looking to **improve health, performance and body composition**

BREAKFAST
- 1 palm-sized portion of whole eggs (~2 eggs)
- 1 fist-sized portion of broccoli, chopped (~1 cup)
- 1 cupped handful of wholegrain toast (~1 slice)
- 1 cupped handful of banana (~1 small)
- 1 thumb of almond butter (~1tbsp)
- Water/green tea/black coffee

LUNCH
- 1 palm-sized portion of chicken (~100g)
- 1 fist-sized portion of spinach (~1 cup)
- ½ cupped handful of sprouted-grain wrap (~½ wrap)
- ½ cupped handful of black beans (~½ cup)
- 1 thumb of pesto (~1tbsp)
- Water/green tea/black coffee

MID-AFTERNOON SUPER SHAKE
- 1 palm-sized portion of vanilla protein (1 scoop)
- 1 fist-sized portion of puréed pumpkin (~1 cup)
- 1 cupped handful of apple (~1 medium)
- 2 thumbs of walnuts (~2tbsp)
- 170ml unsweetened vanilla almond milk
- Ice cubes, cinnamon and vanilla extract as desired

DINNER
- 2 palm-sized portion of wild salmon (~200g)
- 2 fist-sized portion of cauliflower (~1 cup)
- 1 cupped handful of cooked quinoa (~½ cup)
- 1 thumb of extra virgin olive oil (~1tbsp)
- Water

Estimated Nutrition Figures

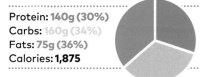

Protein: **140g (30%)**
Carbs: **160g (34%)**
Fats: **75g (36%)**
Calories: **1,875**

Meal Plan 2

For a **woman** who is **lightly active** or looking to **lose bodyweight/fat**

BREAKFAST
- ½ palm-sized portion of whole eggs (~1 egg)
- ½ palm-sized portion of turkey sausage (~½ sausage)
- 1 fist-sized portion of peppers and onions (~1 cup)
- 1 cupped handful of sprouted-grain toast (~1 slice)
- Water/green tea/black coffee

LUNCH
- 1 palm-sized portion of chicken (~100g)
- 1 fist-sized portion of tomatoes and spinach (~1 cup)
- 1 cupped handful of sprouted-grain wrap (1 wrap)
- 1 thumb of guacamole (~1tbsp)
- Water/green tea/black coffee

MID-AFTERNOON SUPER SHAKE
- 1 palm-sized portion of chocolate protein (1 scoop)
- 1 fist-sized portion of spinach (~1 cup)
- 1 cupped handful of banana (~1 small)
- 1 thumb of natural peanut butter (~1tbsp)
- 170ml unsweetened vanilla almond milk
- Ice cubes as desired

DINNER
- 2 palm-sized portions of pork chops (200g)
- 2 fist-sized portions of asparagus (~2 cups)
- 1 thumb of extra virgin olive oil (~1tbsp)
- Water

Estimated Nutrition Figures

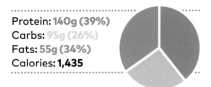

Protein: **140g (39%)**
Carbs: **95g (26%)**
Fats: **55g (34%)**
Calories: **1,435**

Meal Plan 3

For a **woman** who is **highly active** or looking to **build muscle**

BREAKFAST
- 1 palm-sized portion of whole eggs (~2 eggs)
- 1 fist-sized portion of spinach (~1 cup)
- 1 cupped handful of cooked old fashioned oats (~½ cup)
- 1 cupped handful of mixed berries (~½ cup)
- 2 thumbs of slivered almonds (~2tbsp)
- Water/green tea/black coffee

LUNCH
- 1 palm-sized portion of chicken (~100g)
- 1 fist-sized portion of mixed peppers and onions (~1 cup)
- 1 cupped handful of black beans (~½ cup)
- 1 cupped handful of brown and wild rice (~½ cup)
- 2 thumbs of guacamole (~2tbsp)
- Water/green tea/black coffee

MID-AFTERNOON SUPER SHAKE
- 1 palm-sized portion of vanilla protein (1 scoop)
- 1 fist-sized portion of puréed pumpkin (~1 cup)
- 1 cupped handful of apple (~1 medium)
- 2 thumbs of chopped walnuts (~2tbsp)
- 170ml unsweetened vanilla almond milk
- Ice cubes, cinnamon and vanilla extract as desired

DINNER
- 2 palm-sized portions of lean sirloin steak (~200g)
- 2 fist-sized portions of broccoli (~2 cups)
- 2 cupped handfuls potato (~2 small)
- 1 thumb of extra virgin olive oil (~1tbsp)
- Water

Estimated Nutrition Figures

Protein: **150g (28%)**
Carbs: 210g (39%)
Fats: **80g (33%)**
Calories: **2,160**

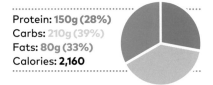

Meal Plan 4

For a **man** looking to **improve health, performance and body composition**

BREAKFAST
- 2 palm-sized portions of whole eggs (~4 eggs)
- 2 fist-sized portions of broccoli, chopped (~2 cups)
- 1 cupped handful of cooked rolled oats (~⅔ cup)
- 1 cupped handful of mixed berries (~⅔ cup)
- 2 thumbs of slivered almonds (~2tbsp)
- Water/green tea/black coffee

LUNCH
- 2 palm-sized portions of chicken (~225g)
- 2 fist-sized portions of mixed peppers and onions, cooked (~2 cups)
- 1 cupped handful of black beans (~⅔ cup)
- 1 cupped handful of cooked brown and wild rice (~⅔ cup)
- 2 thumbs of guacamole (~2tbsp)
- Water/green tea/black coffee

MID-AFTERNOON SUPER SHAKE
- 1 palm-sized portions of strawberry protein (1 scoop)
- 1 fist-sized portion of spinach (~1 cup)
- 1 cupped handfuls of frozen mixed berries (~⅔ cup)
- 1 thumbs of walnuts (~1tbsp)
- 170ml unsweetened vanilla almond milk
- Ice cubes as desired

DINNER
- 2 palm-sized portions of lean sirloin steak (~225g)
- 2 fist-sized portions of asparagus (~2 cups)
- 2 cupped handfuls of potato (~1 large)
- 1 thumb of extra virgin olive oil (~1tbsp)
- 1 thumb of butter (~1tbsp)
- Water

Estimated Nutrition Figures

Protein: **200g (32%)**
Carbs: 230g (37%)
Fats: **85g (31%)**
Calories: **2,485**

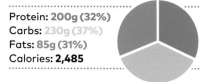

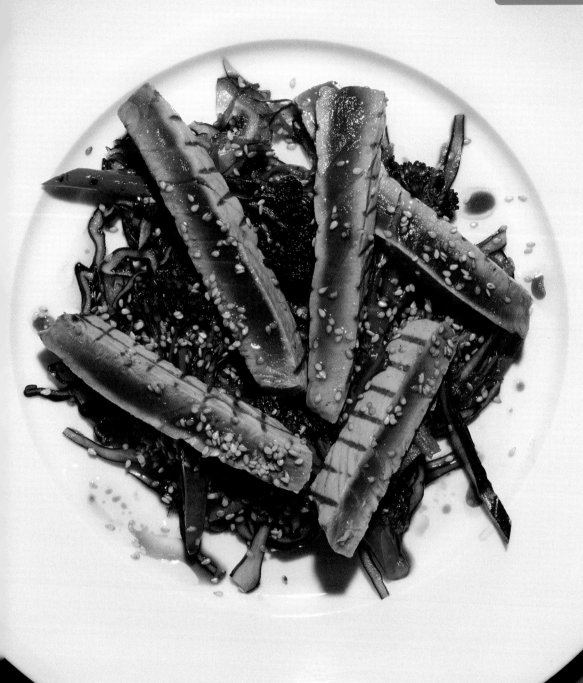

Meal Plan 5

For a **man** who is **lightly active** or looking to **lose body weight/fat**

BREAKFAST
- 2 palm-sized portions of whole eggs (~4 eggs)
- 2 fist-sized portions of mixed peppers and onions (~2 cups)
- 1 cupped handful of cooked rolled oats (~⅔ cup)
- 1 cupped handful of mixed berries (~⅔ cup)
- 1 thumb of chopped walnuts (~1tbsp)
- Water/green tea/black coffee

LUNCH
- 2 palm-sized portions of chicken (~225g)
- 2 fist-sized portions of mixed greens, chopped carrots and cucumbers (~2 cups)
- 1 cupped handful of black beans (~⅔ cup)
- 1 thumb of guacamole (~1tbsp)
- Water/green tea/black coffee

MID-AFTERNOON SUPER SHAKE
- 1 palm-sized portion of chocolate protein (1 scoop)
- 1 fist-sized portion of spinach (~1 cup)
- 1 cupped handful of sweet dark cherries (~⅔ cup)
- 1 thumb of almonds (~1tbsp)
- 170ml unsweetened vanilla almond milk
- Ice cubes as desired

DINNER
- 2 palm-sized portions of wild salmon (~225g)
- 2 fist-sized portions of courgette (~2 cups)
- 1 cupped handful of sweet potato (~1 medium)
- 1 thumb of extra virgin olive oil (~1tbsp)
- 1 thumb of butter (~1tbsp)
- Water

Estimated Nutrition Figures

Protein: **185g (35%)**
Carbs: 160g (30%)
Fats: **80g (35%)**
Calories: **2,100**

Meal Plan 6

For a **man** who is **highly active** or looking to **build muscle**

BREAKFAST
- 1 palm-sized portion of whole eggs (~2 eggs)
- 1 palm-sized portion of chicken sausage (~1 sausage)
- 2 fist-sized portions of spinach (~2 cups)
- 2 cupped handfuls of wholegrain toast (~2 slices)
- 1 cupped handful of banana (1 medium)
- 2 thumbs of peanut butter (~2 thumbs)
- Water/green tea/black coffee

LUNCH
- 2 palm-sized portions of chicken (~225g)
- 2 fist-sized portions of mixed peppers and onions (~2 cups)
- 1 cupped handful of black beans (~2/3 cup)
- 2 cupped handfuls of cooked brown and wild rice (~1⅓ cups)
- 2 thumbs of guacamole (~2tbsp)
- Water/green tea/black coffee

MID-AFTERNOON SUPER SHAKE
- 2 palm-sized portions of strawberry protein (2 scoops)
- 2 fist-sized portions of spinach (~2 cups)
- 1 cupped handful of banana (~1 medium)
- 1 cupped handful of blueberries (~2/3 cup)
- 3 thumbs of almonds (~3 tbsp)
- 340ml unsweetened vanilla almond milk
- Ice cubes as desired

DINNER
- 2 palm-sized portions of pork (~225g)
- 2 fist-sized portions of green beans (~2 cups)
- 2 cupped handfuls of cooked quinoa (~1⅓ cups)
- 2 thumbs of extra virgin olive oil (~2tbsp)
- Water

Estimated Nutrition Figures

Protein: **255g (31%)**
Carbs: 305g (37%)
Fats: **115g (32%)**
Calories: **3,275**

You and your gut

The gut is known as your "second brain" with good reason, and taking better care of it will pay big health and happiness rewards

The old saying goes that "you are what you eat". But a more accurate version would be "you are what you absorb". The food you eat has an enormous effect on your health and well-being, from how easily you lose or gain weight to your risk of certain illnesses and diseases. What is not so well understood, but just as important, is the impact of how you eat and how this affects nutrient absorption.

Research shows listening to different types of music, eating from coloured plates and even the weight of cutlery can all affect the speed and amount you eat, as well as your meal enjoyment. But it's not just external factors at play: the digestive system is highly sensitive to signals coming from your brain, and your physiological and psychological state at mealtimes has a significant impact on how well you digest food and absorb nutrients.

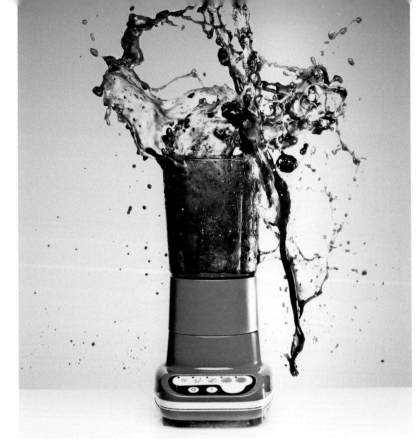

The digestion process

The digestive system is composed of the mouth, oesophagus, stomach, small intestine, large intestine (or gut) and rectum. Digestion starts in the mouth, with the enzymes in your saliva that begin to break down food, but most of the action occurs in your stomach.

That's where enzymes reduce the larger pieces of food into smaller components. Proteases break down proteins into amino acids; amylases break down carbs into simple sugars; and lipases break down fats into fatty acids.

These nutrients are then absorbed through the wall of the small intestine into the bloodstream where they travel through the circulatory system until they get to where they're needed. Any nutrients that aren't immediately needed are stored or excreted.

Stress and digestion

You've probably heard of the "fight, flight or freeze" response, which is how the body responds to danger for survival, known scientifically as the sympathetic nervous system. We also have the parasympathetic nervous system, which is the "rest and digest" side to the system.

These two parts of the nervous system work like traffic lights: when one system is "on" or green, the other is "off" or red. They can't both be green at the same time (otherwise there'll be chaos).

What's this got to do with eating and your gut? A lot, actually! Because the two systems can't run simultaneously, that means when you're stressed it is very difficult to digest food properly. Your appetite is suppressed, the movement of food through your digestive system slows, and blood flow is directed away from your digestive tract to your limbs to help you escape or fight off the perceived danger.

Chronic stress

While we no longer face that "quick, run, there's a tiger!" type of acute stress, many of us suffer from long-term or "chronic" stress that seems an inevitable part of modern life (it's not inevitable, and we'll get to that soon!).

Chronic stress is really bad for your health. It depletes essential nutrients and impairs the body's repair, growth and recovery processes; it causes more of what you eat to be poorly digested; and it can create impairments in the gut that trigger allergies, bloating and autoimmune disorders such as IBS.

It also diverts our attention and energy to what's stressing us and away from more beneficial activities. Prolonged periods of stress can drive us to use food as a distraction or escape, and you're less likely to be aware of what and how much you're eating, increasing the chances of overeating and making matters worse.

Quick tip

Your gut and your brain are very closely linked and your digestive system shuts down when you're stressed. Eating in a stressed state reduces how well your body is able to digest the food you eat and absorb nutrients from it, increases the risk of overeating and weight gain, and isn't enjoyable – in short, it sucks! The good news is that there's an antidote to stressful eating and it can make you leaner and happier! Turn the page to discover more about mindful eating.

Mealtime mindfulness

Here's why being more "present" when you eat can make you leaner and happier!

We've mentioned "mindfulness" and "mindful eating" briefly already, so here's what it means and why being mindful during meals makes a big difference to your health and happiness.

Mindfulness is simply the practice of paying attention (in a non-judgemental way) to an activity. It's a very effective method to manage stress: one study found regular mindfulness meditation actually changes the structure of the brain, creating more neural connections, which might protect us from depression and dementia.

Ultimately, being more mindful gives you a different perspective on your thoughts and feelings and helps you approach situations in a calmer, more thoughtful way. And being mindful when eating can have a positive impact on your physical and mental health, without requiring too much effort!

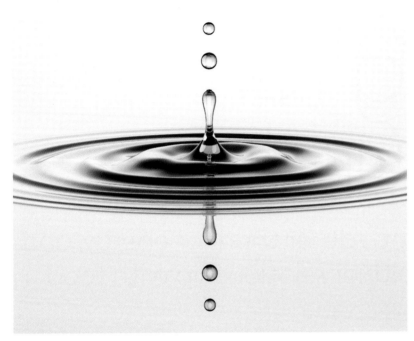

The mindfulness connection

When you eat mindfully you pay attention to the appearance, texture and taste of your food, and your body's hunger signals. It takes time for your brain to register signals from your stomach's stretch receptors, so mindful eating can prevent overeating by slowing you down and making you more aware of how you're feeling (regularly overeating can blunt your body's fullness signals and contribute to weight gain). Mindfulness can also enhance the pleasure you derive from food, so you're less likely to overeat because you've taken time to really enjoy your meal. Being more mindful also makes it easier to eat a wider variety of foods, and being non-judgemental makes you open to trying new foods. This is important because you might be missing out on something you'll really like, and the more varied your diet the lower your risk of any nutrient deficiencies.

Eat mindfully with ease!

You don't need any special equipment or apps to begin mindful eating – in fact, the fewer distractions you have the better! Here's how to get started:

1. Turn off the TV and put away your phone. We're so used to watching or reading while eating that this might feel difficult at first, so really focus on the colours and smells on your plate.

Quick tip

Eating when distracted reduces your enjoyment of food and increases the risk of overeating and emotional eating. But practising slow, mindful eating, chewing every mouthful properly, will heighten your enjoyment of food, improve digestion and help prevent overeating!

2. Sit at a table. This will help you focus on the food in front of you and re-emphasises that mealtimes are an important activity, not a chore to be squeezed in where possible.

3. Start small. Being mindful at mealtimes takes time and practice and you will get distracted. Begin by aiming to take just one mindful mouthful per meal. Here's how:

Take a moment to look at the food on the plate, noticing the smells, colours and textures.

Pick up a forkful or spoonful and take a moment to notice the qualities of the food.

Take the bite and chew slowly, noticing the different flavours and textures and how they change as you chew.

Put down your cutlery. This helps you focus on swallowing this mouthful before starting the next.

After you swallow, be aware of the food moving to your stomach and how it affects your level of hunger.

If you are new to mindful eating you can continue eating in this way, or return to your old eating habits. But do try to add in an extra mindful mouthful each day until you eat a full mindful meal.

Just one mindful meal or snack a day will improve your relationship with food and help you listen to and understand your body better.

Eating for pleasure!

Eat for enjoyment, rather than for energy, and you'll forge a healthier relationship with food

Food plays a central role in our lives, not just as our source of energy and nutrients, but in how it makes us feel. Eating a wide variety of foods you enjoy, in a relaxed environment and in good company, is vital to your well-being because through meals we socialise, celebrate and connect with others. So when we talk about a "balanced diet" it's not just about nutrients – it's also about perspective!

Yes, we all have a responsibility to our future selves to take care of ourselves now, which means having a healthy diet. But we must also remember that we live social and emotional lives and food is a big part of that.

One problem is the highly stylised food photography on social media of "clean foods" or "clean eating" meals. This can distort the relationship between the foods we should eat and our long-term health and happiness.

Dietitians and nutritionists agree that the quality of a diet is measured over the long term by a good balance of nutrients *and* deriving pleasure from eating, not from looking at each meal in isolation with a "good' or "bad" judgement.

Pause for pleasure

On p44 we explained that eating well 80% of the time is a fantastic target for greater health and happiness, and a great way to hit that target regularly is to start thinking about foods not as "good" or "bad", but as "nutrient-dense" or "pleasurable", both of which are positive terms.

Ideally, we'll eat meals that are both nourishing and pleasurable: a bowl of soup may contain several servings of vegetables as well as being just the thing to warm and comfort us on a cold day. But finding that balance across a meal, or across the week, is the aim. Remember, it's the bigger picture of your food choices that matters. If, after checking in with yourself, you decide that you want something just for pleasure, then go for it and allow yourself to enjoy it!

Here's where mindfulness helps: take your time to enjoy the smell, texture and flavour of

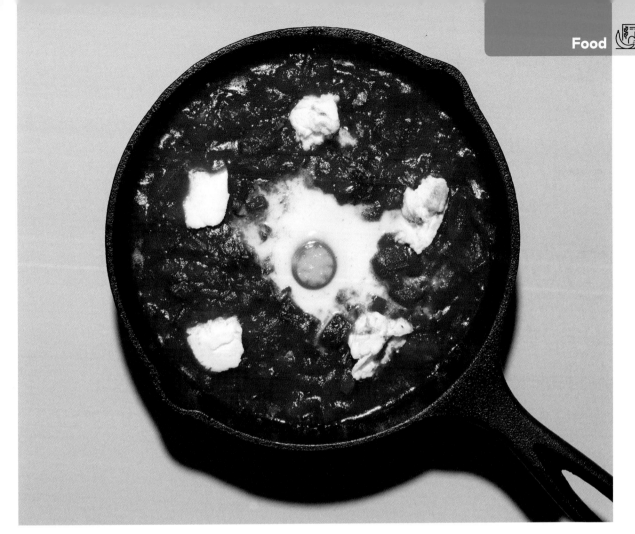

the food completely. There's no point in eating a pleasure food and then feeling guilty about it!

The problem with feeling guilty about food, aside from feeling miserable, is it sets you up for "black and white" thinking in other areas of your life too. The "all or nothing" approach we discussed earlier always leads to nothing, and this type of thinking triggers the idea that if something isn't "perfect" then it's worthless. You might think to yourself "I've blown it" and then lose motivation to exercise, or fill in your journal or do any other beneficial activities you'd planned.

Quick tip

Some foods are good for the soul and it's really important to know you can eat and enjoy them without suffering any negative emotion. This is where being mindful before and during meals is helpful for improving your health and happiness. If you are still prone to overeating then turn the page to discover the tried-and-tested strategies to beat bingeing for good!

Food and your mood

Interestingly, letting go of guilt and enjoying your food has other beneficial consequences. Research shows that when we're in a better mood we tend to make healthier food choices, while negative moods do the opposite. So, feeling guilty about eating something could create a self-defeating vicious cycle of binge eating and negative feelings.

The other issue with food guilt is the well-known experience that the more you restrict something, the more you tell yourself you can't have it, the more you crave it. You become obsessed with the thing you cannot have, increasing the likelihood that at some point you will gorge on it. Research suggests non-restrictive eaters – people who allow themselves to eat what they want – have fewer obsessive food thoughts and are less likely to binge. Now there's some food for thought!

How to stop overeating!

It can be easy to eat too much despite not wanting to and it makes losing fat tough. Here's why it happens, and how you can stop it

Whether it's a birthday, a holiday, socialising with friends or just a Friday night with a takeaway pizza, all of us at some point eat too much. But for some of us this happens more often than we'd like. Here we'll look at some of the main reasons that can trigger over-eating, and then we'll provide some really simple strategies you can use to overcome them.

FACTOR 1

Your prehistoric brain

The first thing to understand about overeating is that most of it isn't your fault – at least, not consciously. Evolution has ensured that our brains pay a lot of attention to food; that our brains prefer sweet, fatty and savoury foods that are high in energy; and that we tend to eat more rather than less, in case a famine is around the corner.

This was a life-saving strategy until very recently in human history. But we now live in a world where food, especially processed food high in calories but low in nutrients, is tasty, cheap and accessible, and hard to quit eating once you start. Food manufacturers know what our hungry brains like and purposely make processed foods that appeal to them.

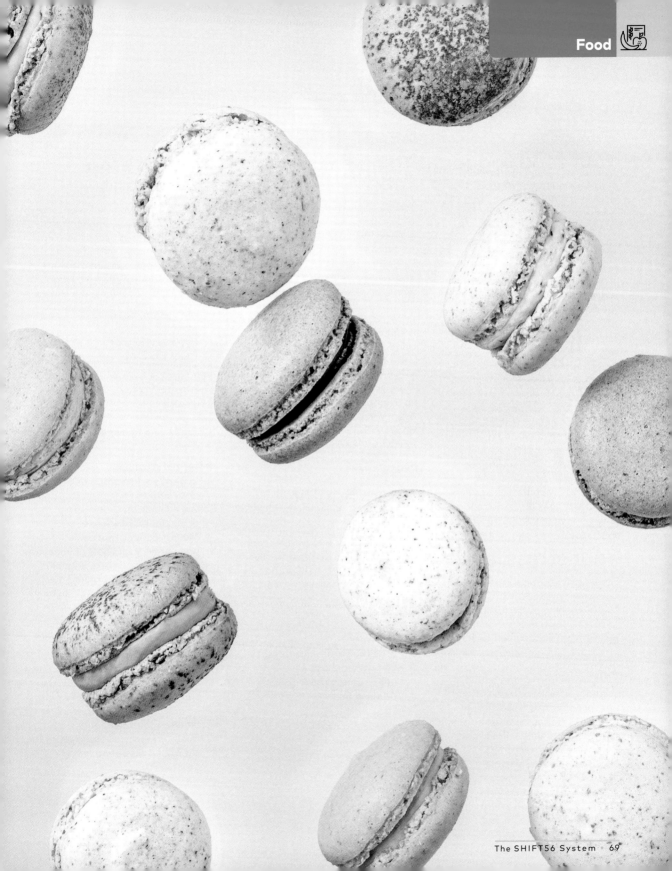

FACTOR 2
Your food triggers

We make hundreds of food decisions a day, but we aren't aware of most of them. We rarely consciously choose what and how to eat. Instead, we tend to go on autopilot and rely on routines, habits and what's easiest.

We eat in our cars, on the train, walking to work, at our desks and on the go, usually without stopping and thinking about it. When we see or smell food we just grab it and eat it, and we rarely slow down, sit down and experience it mindfully with full awareness. We're often mentally or physically tired, which makes it even harder to make smart food choices, which is why the advice on achieving mealtime mindfulness (p64) is so important.

And if you're a woman your natural hormonal fluctuations may affect your hunger, appetite and ability to control your eating.

FACTOR 3
Your stress levels

Stress and emotional well-being are the two other big factors behind overeating.

Most of us feel some level of stress in our lives, as well as difficult emotions such as loneliness, anxiety, guilt and fatigue. We may feel over-stimulated from stress or under-stimulated from boredom. Food is a very effective "medication" for stress, difficult emotions and over- or under-stimulation. At least, it is temporarily.

Then, of course, we might feel more stressed or worse after we've overeaten. And so the cycle begins again.

FACTOR 4
Your self-imposed food rules

Many people try to "fix" overeating with a strict diet or eating rules such as "No food after 7pm" or "No sugar ever again".

Unfortunately, as you now know, these restrictions backfire. You soon resent following such rules, or feel deprived. If you've reduced what you eat dramatically, your body responds by turning up the appetite signals and attention to food cues, so food becomes really, really appealing.

Eventually, people go right back to overeating and then they feel even worse. The cycle repeats, over and over, and each time it becomes harder and harder to break.

FACTOR 5
Your regular routine

We all have routines and for many of us, there are certain times when we are more likely to overeat. These are the most common...

- Weekends
- Evenings
- After work
- Parties and other social events
- After the kids have – finally – gone to bed
- Watching TV

How to stop overeating

Looking back over the list of factors above, two things jump out as the biggest causes of overeating on a day-to-day basis: eating quickly and eating while distracted. So there are two really simple first steps you could take to deal with these:

- Slow down the speed at which you eat.
- Pay attention to the foods you are eating.

Here are some other contributing factors and some strategies you could use to overcome them.

Contributing factor #1
You see "food cues" everywhere

Potential strategies
- Look at your environment and routines to see where you can adjust, control and/or eliminate those cues.
- Make it easier to eat healthy foods and harder to get hold of unhealthy ones. So if you have a "trigger" food, don't keep it in your house.

Contributing factor #2
You fall into automatic behaviours without realising

Potential strategies
- Slow down. Pause before you make choices. Ask yourself, "Is this the smartest choice I can make right now? What might be better?"
- Sit at a table to eat and focus as much as possible on the actual act of eating.

Contributing factor #3
You always eat too quickly

Potential strategies
- Eat slowly and chew your food for longer.
- Put down your cutlery between mouthfuls.
- Take a breath between each bite.
- Try to really taste and savour the food.

Contributing factor #4
You turn to food when stressed or emotional

Potential strategies
- Take a few deep breaths before you make a food choice or start eating.
- Ask yourself, "Am I feeling hungry right now?" Pause and identify whether you might be thinking or experiencing another feeling.
- Seek help with managing stress and emotions from a therapist or counsellor.

Contributing factor #5
You impose strict eating rules on yourself

Potential strategies
- Recognise that restrictive rules, or following a strict diet, is not a solution to overeating – indeed it may even increase and worsen your overeating habit in the long run.

Other strategies
As we discussed earlier in this chapter, it's not helpful to label individual foods with rigid moral labels such as "good versus bad" or "clean versus cheating". Instead use categories such as...

- "eat more often" or "eat less often"
- "works well for me" or "doesn't work well for me"
- "makes me feel better" or "makes me feel worse"

Instead of using external rules, work on learning your own internal signals of hunger and fullness, and don't feel failure, frustration or shame after an overeating episode: treat yourself with compassion. Look at each overeating episode as an opportunity to learn more about your triggers so that you can keep finding better ways to overcome them next time.

Start to ask yourself more questions about your daily and weekly routines and identify your triggers, then write down some solutions to overcome them. For instance, where and when are you less likely to overeat? What works well about those situations? Can you do or get more of that? Conversely, where and when are you more likely to overeat? How can you disrupt those situations or do something differently?

Keep moving forwards!
As you learn to change your habits you'll make mistakes. That's normal! Changing behaviours takes time so if you do overeat don't beat yourself up: this will only make it worse. Try to use these responses instead.

- Stay positive! Focus on what you're doing well and the positive choices you've been making. Most of the time, we're doing better than we realise!
- Recognise it's normal. Many people struggle with overeating. You're not bad or broken!
- Keep learning, and notice what situations and factors make it easier for you to make wiser food choices.
- Think like a scientist! Take notes about what caused you to overeat and what occurred when you did. Analyse that info and look for patterns to identify strategies for the future.
- Reboot asap! Wipe the slate clean and start again, immediately. Every time will get a little bit easier.

Quick tip

The biggest factors behind overeating are speed, distraction and stress. So slow down, breathe and pay attention! Choose natural whole foods such as fruits and vegetables, which make you feel healthy, satisfied and energetic, and try to eat until sated, not stuffed! Take the time to listen to your body's natural hunger and fullness signals, and appreciate the simple act of sitting down and savouring every mouthful.

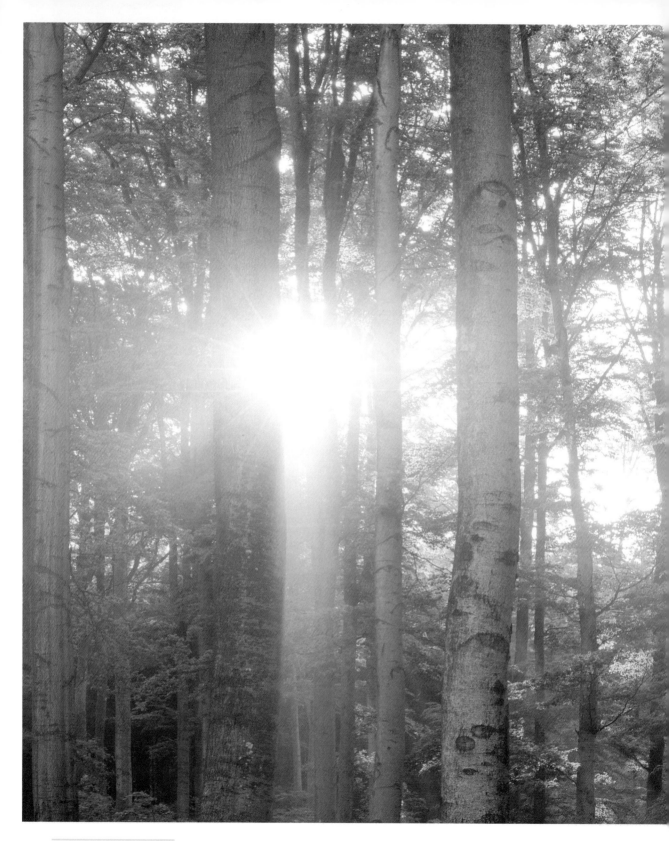

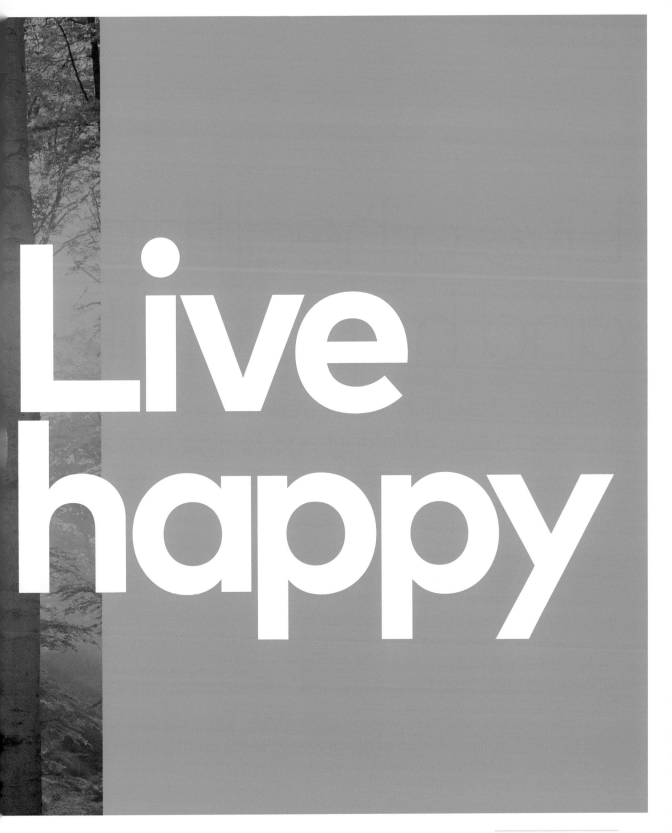

Live happy

Live a healthier and happier life!

Making a few simple lifestyle changes is all it takes to start looking and feeling fantastic

There are 168 hours in each week. Once you take out about three hours of exercise and, say, 10 hours for cooking and eating, that leaves 155 hours. That's a lot of time! The point is that while exercising and eating well have a big contribution on how good you look and feel, what you do in those other 155 hours each week also has a huge impact on the quality of your life. Take sleep. Getting enough quality sleep is hugely important to your mental and physical health, and even a single night of poor sleep drastically affects how you think, feel, look and perform the next day.

In this chapter, you'll discover the proven ways to improve both the quality and duration of your sleep, as well as some really quick and easy habit changes that will make you look and feel better than ever! Then you'll find out about your SHIFT56 Journal, which makes it incredibly easy for you to take back control of your health and happiness!

Chapter Contents

3 myths of happiness

Make sure you're looking for happiness in the right places by avoiding these feel-good fallacies

Modern life can be tough and sometimes it feels as if true happiness is always out of reach. That makes it tempting to try to force happiness to happen by seeking shortcuts. These may make us feel better temporarily, but they're very unlikely to address the underlying issues that prevent us from living the genuinely happier life we want.

Here are three of the most common myths people think can create happiness – and why they don't work. On the next page we'll explain the really simple strategies that will make you feel better for good – starting right now!

MYTH 1

"I'll be happy when I have the perfect body"

Believing you'll only be happy when you have the "perfect body" is one of the most damaging types of internal pressure, and thinking like this can make you really unhappy. Mainly because the perfect body doesn't exist.

That doesn't mean it's impossible to make a big difference to how you look naked – you can! – but it's very hard to be objective about our own bodies, no matter how much progress we've made. It's really important to shift that mindset into feeling happy by taking control of your health and fitness today through exercise, eating well and your journal. That's how you'll find immediate and lasting happiness, rather than obsessing over an outcome that's impossible to achieve.

"I'll be happy when I'm successful"

Believing you'll only be happy when you are perceived as successful or important by other people can damage your hopes of happiness as much as chasing the perfect body.

First, linking your sense of self-worth to the opinions of others is a waste of time. Do you "grade" family, friends or colleagues based on their job, or how much money or success they have? No, so it's unlikely anyone whose opinion you respect is doing the same to you!

Second, if someone does appear to judge you they're not somebody whose opinion you should care about. Nobody other than you can truly understand or appreciate everything you've done and everything you are, so any negative opinion you receive is never an accurate reflection of reality.

"I can spend my way to happiness"

Treating yourself to a new item of clothing or gadget might make you feel a bit better, but this enjoyment won't last long. Indeed a "I will spend myself happy" attitude may result in greater unhappiness over time. Our levels of happiness are fairly stable and while a new car or dress or shoes might make you feel a little happier for a while, you soon grow accustomed to the new item and start looking for more products or status symbols to give yourself another boost. Before long you end up on a "treat treadmill", constantly chasing the next luxury item that will make you happy.

A better strategy is to work on some of the positive habit changes we suggest on the next page. Putting them into practice will lead to higher happiness levels – day in, day out!

10 tools for building better life habits

Lose weight and live happier with these smart, simple and sustainable lifestyle adjustments

Almost all our behaviours take the form of a habit. Some of these regular routines are great: brushing your teeth is important for avoiding a toothless old age; and making your partner a cup of tea first thing demonstrates appreciation and deepens your bond. But other habits are not so beneficial: hitting the snooze button every morning means you always end up rushing and arrive at work already stressed.

So we all have lots of habits that either enhance or impede our lives, but the good news is there's always the opportunity to break unhelpful habits and create new, beneficial ones.

Establishing good habits reduces the number of decisions you have to make each day, freeing up brainpower for more important tasks. It also reduces the amount of firefighting you have to do fixing problems created by bad habits. Research shows there are some habits that bring a wealth of physical and mental health benefits – and you'll find them over the page!

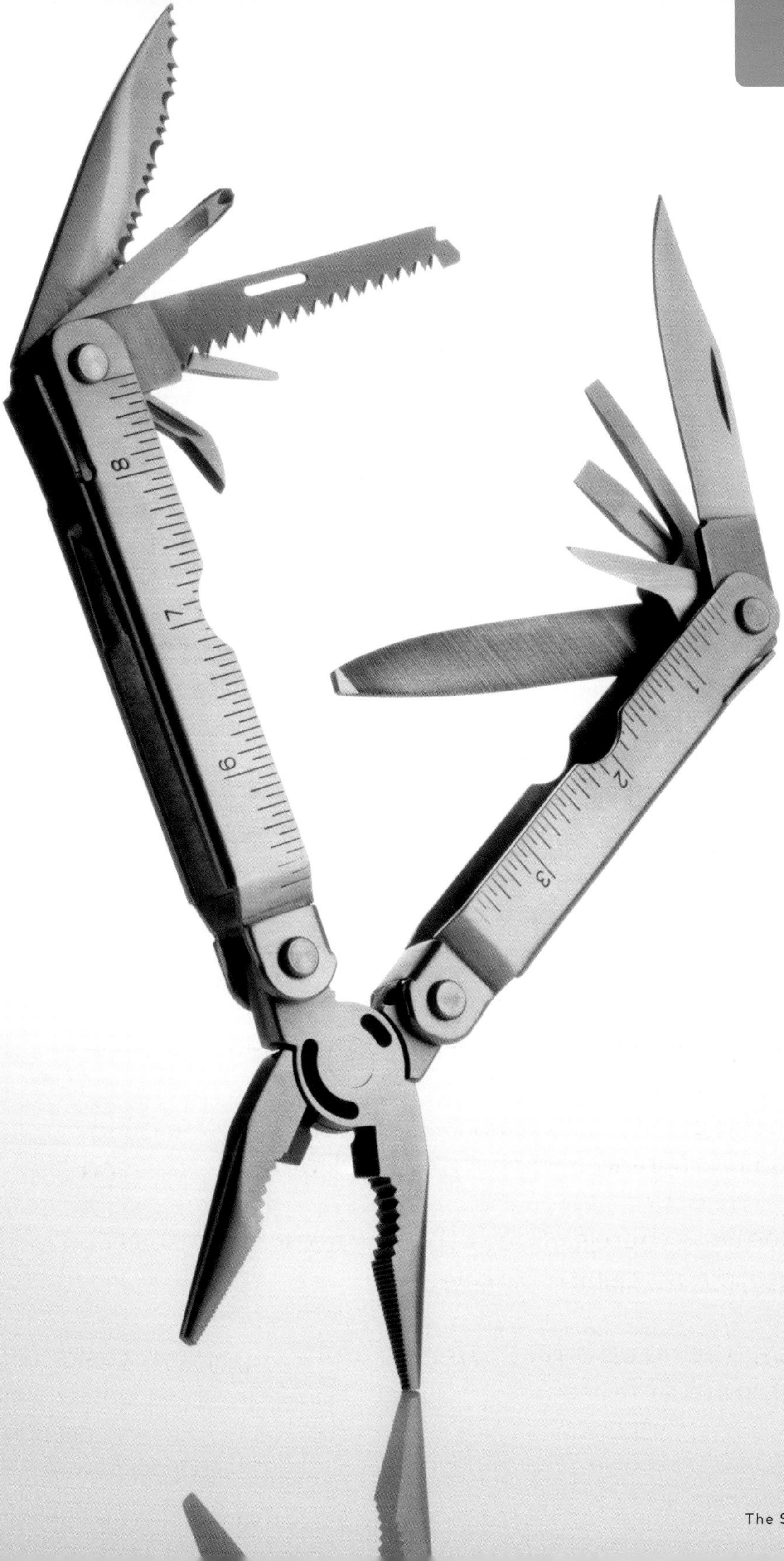
8
7
6
1
2
3

ONE
Be more active

The physical and mental benefits of exercise are so numerous and well established that if exercise were a pill, we'd all be trying to stockpile it. As well as helping you lose body fat and increase lean body mass, exercise also protects the long-term health of the brain in two main ways.

Aerobic activity, such as running, swimming and cycling, increases blood flow to the brain, which brings with it oxygen and nutrients that the brain needs to stay in good working order.

Resistance training, such as bodyweight exercise or lifting dumbbells increases the production of compounds in the brain that protect nerve cells from dying, and promotes the growth of new neural connections. A better-connected brain is faster and more efficient and this extra connectivity, if continued over a long period of time, can protect against the loss of brain volume as we age.

But physical activity isn't only running or doing press-ups: the habit of simply moving more often is linked to longevity and better brain function as we age. If you can start getting into the habit of going for a 20- or 30-minute walk every lunchtime you will make significant strides to improve your health and well-being.

TWO
Eat more veg

From a nutrition perspective eating more greens is probably the single most important new habit you can forge to enhance your health. Veggies are packed with vitamins, minerals, fibre and other compounds such as phytochemicals that have numerous health-boosting qualities. As we explained on p52 you should be eating a fist-sized portion of veggies with every meal if you're a woman, and two if you're a man, and this should be the absolute minimum.

It's also important to eat a wide range of veggies, because each type and colour contains different combinations of essential nutrients. If you don't like certain vegetables, experiment with different cooking methods or adding different spices or oils to make them more palatable.

THREE
Drink more water

Staying hydrated has repeatedly been shown to improve physical and mental well-being and performance. Research has found people encouraged to drink more water felt less fatigued, had better focus and improved mood, and felt less tired – all factors that promote a sense of well-being. Aim for around two litres a day, but more if you exercise or if it's hot and humid, and carry a water bottle around with you so it's easy to keep drinking all day long.

FOUR
Be more mindful

Getting into the habit of focusing your attention on what's happening in the here and now can lower stress levels, stop you feeling overwhelmed, and improve productivity. A regular mindfulness practice can also reduce inflammation, induce calm and even protect brain health. If you're new to the practice of mindfulness, start with just being more mindful at mealtimes, as we discussed on p64.

FIVE
Be more grateful

It is so easy to get into the habit of complaining about the things that we don't have or that have gone wrong. It is important to face certain realities, but we need to be careful not to overemphasise the negatives to the detriment of all the good things we have going on.

Simply writing down one thing you're grateful for each day as part of your SHIFT56 Journal, which we will get to in more detail on p90, is a genuinely powerful tool for rebalancing your attention and focusing more on the good things in life.

SIX
Make connections

It isn't being dramatic to say loneliness kills. Despite a dizzying array of "social" media platforms many people find they are more isolated and disconnected than ever. Loneliness increases your risk of heart attack, depression and cognitive decline. When people look back on their lives in old age one of the biggest regrets is neglecting relationships, and research shows the people who live longest have cultivated close relationships and are part of stable communities.

Get into the habit of prioritising your relationships. Even if you have to schedule phone calls or make arrangements weeks in advance, it's worth the effort because in-person contact with people who matter to you pays huge dividends to your well-being.

SEVEN
Open up more

There are serious physiological consequences to bottling up your feelings. Not only does it increase dissatisfaction and unhappiness, but holding on to negative emotions can increase inflammation in the body, which is associated with a number of health risks from depression to heart disease. Get into the habit of saying how you feel as soon as you can – you'll be protecting your health, as well as helping prevent the resentment and misunderstandings that harm relationships. If you find it difficult to say how you feel or are in the habit of putting on a brave face, talking to an impartial professional can give you the skills and confidence to be more open.

EIGHT
Be more organised

Are you always running for the train or ignoring bills until they're sent in red ink? Does the word "deadline" conjure up images of caffeine-fuelled all-nighters? If that sounds like you, you need to get more organised, because doing so will reduce your everyday stress levels to make becoming healthier and happier far easier. It's as simple as putting out your work clothes the night before, or planning and cooking your meals in advance, and we have plenty more advice on how to get on top of your life at shift56.com.

 Quick tip

Habit change is hard, even when we know it will do us the power of good in the long run, and it takes time and effort to break established routines and rewire your brain to the better way of doing things. Start small, breaking the beneficial habit down into smaller steps and take just one step at a time. And give yourself a break – it's not easy but it will be worth it!

NINE
Get a hobby

For many of us work is something we have to do to enjoy the rest of our lives. Maybe one day you could see whether your personal and professional interests could overlap, but for now it's vital to remember that your job is not your identity, nor is it the extent of your capabilities. Explore that hobby that's always interested you: learn to dance, play an instrument, learn a language, try something you think you'll love. Don't have enough time? Watch an hour less TV a night and now you do! Your new hobby will give you far more satisfaction and ultimately lead to greater happiness.

TEN
Sort your sleep

Skimping on sleep will make you tired, unproductive, depressed, fat and sick – and it'll shorten your life. Developing better bedtime and sleep habits will make a phenomenal difference to your life. Find out what you can do on p86.

Hormones, health and happiness

How good you look and feel is determined by your hormones – here's how to get them working for you

Imagine a telephone network that stretches all over the world. Everyone can call everyone else. And you can call several people at once. Or they can call you. And 100 of your closest friends simultaneously. If you can imagine how complicated that might be, you can start to understand a bit more about how your hormones work! They control all our important bodily functions, and they have lots of interconnected effects, so it's vital to maintain a balance if you're going to be healthier and happier. And that's easier than it might sound – turn the page to find out how!

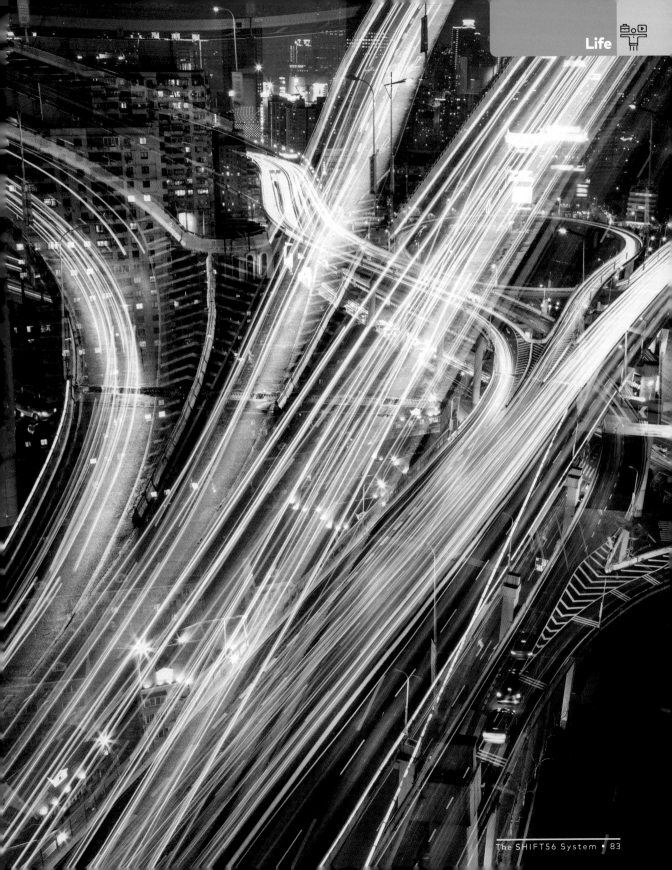

Hormones, and other cell signalling molecules known as cytokines, send messages around our bodies like air traffic controllers organising the skies around them. These messages control all our physiological and metabolic activities, including...

- digesting and absorbing nutrients
- hunger and appetite
- sleep and wakefulness
- growth and development
- tissue recovery and repair
- thinking, memory and mood
- stress response
- reproduction and sexual health
- balancing our fluids, salts and minerals (which also includes blood pressure)

And, just like a large phone network or busy airport, hormones need to work together in a coordinated, highly organised way.

What are the key hormones?

Endocrinology – the science of hormones – is a relatively new field of research and we are discovering new chemical signals and messengers all the time. Also, most hormones come in more than one form and have several jobs. For instance, oestrogen governs women's fertililty, but also helps control inflammation and maintain brain function. Here are some of the most important hormones and what they do.

Hormones involved in digestion, hunger, and appetite

Insulin is released when we eat carbohydrates. It helps to balance blood sugar and move nutrients into cells.

Glucagon is secreted when we haven't eaten in a while. It helps break down stored glucose (sugar).

Leptin is secreted mostly in fat cells and helps tell our body how much energy we have, mostly in the form of stored body fat.

Cholecystokinin (CCK) is released in the small intestine when we eat protein and fat to help us feel full.

Hormones involved in mood and cognition

Serotonin is a "feelgood" hormone that calms us and helps us sleep.

Dopamine is part of our "reward" system that encourages us to explore, take risks, focus on challenges and try new things.

Oxytocin is an anti-stress hormone that's secreted when we are feeling safe and connected to others.

Hormones involved in stress response

Cortisol is released in normal daily

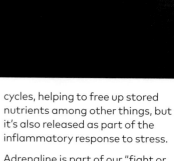

cycles, helping to free up stored nutrients among other things, but it's also released as part of the inflammatory response to stress.

Adrenaline is part of our "fight or flight" system that quickly frees up energy for responding to danger.

Hormones involved in reproduction and fertility

Both men and women have these sex hormones, but in different amounts.

Oestrogen and progesterone organise women's menstrual cycles and sexual development.

Testosterone is men's main sexual and reproductive hormone. It's also important for building muscle.

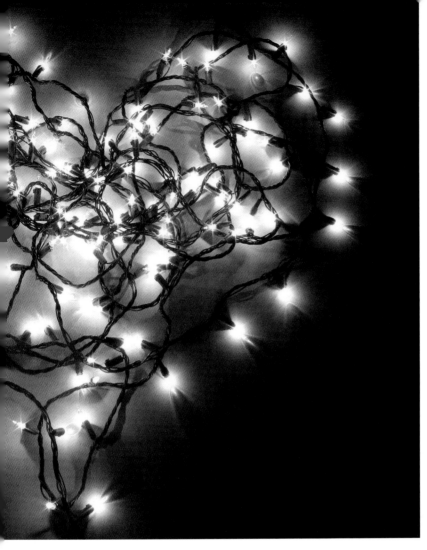

Symptoms of hormonal imbalances can be very varied, but typically include changes in appetite, mood, memory, sleep or energy levels; changes to your libido or sexual function; differences in how much body fat is stored and where; or difficulty losing weight or gaining lean muscle. For women, changes to reproductive and sexual hormones may show up as irregular or absent periods, pelvic and breast pain, infertility, and/or loss of libido.

If you have any concerns, before you self-diagnose using the internet, go and see your GP. Many of the major hormones can be easily tested using blood, urine or saliva tests.

Keeping hormones healthy

We can influence some of these hormonal changes with simple lifestyle habits, such as managing stress; getting good-quality sleep, adequate exercise and recovery; losing excess body fat; building lean muscle mass; eating a balanced and varied diet; limiting alcohol intake and not smoking.

Hormonal balance

We want our hormones to be well coordinated – available at the right times, for the right reasons, in the right amounts. Many hormones have natural rhythms, such as the daily rhythm of cortisol (which normally peaks in the early morning and slowly declines throughout the day) or the monthly cycle of menstruation.

You may have heard that certain hormones are "bad", but our bodies are complex systems with natural variations, and all hormones have important jobs. For instance, we want insulin to go up after we eat a meal with carbohydrates because it helps shuttle nutrients into our cells. However, at other times, we want insulin to be lower. Likewise, we want cortisol to go up in the early morning to release stored fuel for energy while we sleep, and to control inflammation in the early stages of injury. But at other times, like before bed, we want cortisol to be relatively low so we can get to sleep!

Hormonal imbalance

The most common cause of a hormonal imbalance is stress, but there are other factors, such as normal ageing; environmental toxins; having too much or not enough body fat; major dietary changes; pregnancy and lactation; serious injury or illness; drug and alcohol use; or medication.

Quick tip

The hormone system is complex but designed to keep your body performing optimally through a continuous feedback loop that tweaks levels to maintain balance. Stress is the most common cause of a hormone imbalance, which can have many negative short- and long-term health impacts. Luckily some very simple lifestyle changes – which we outline over the next few pages – can help keep your hormone levels healthy!

Sleep sounder tonight!

Get high-quality restorative sleep every night to transform how you look and feel

There's supposed to be something very impressive about getting by with very little sleep. We hear highly successful people who get by with only four or five hours a night described as "superhuman". But there is nothing big or clever about surviving on very little sleep. For people who are not natural "short-sleepers" (thought to be just 2% of the population), poor and disturbed sleep is a serious problem. Indeed, a recent UK poll found that only 50% of us are happy with the amount of sleep we get.

Poor sleep has serious consequences for your physical health – it's associated with increased risk of obesity and heart disease – and your mental health. It increases the risk of depression and mood disorders, and impairs decision making, concentration, communication and language skills, among many other problems. But we have the solutions, so read on to learn how to sleep better – starting tonight!

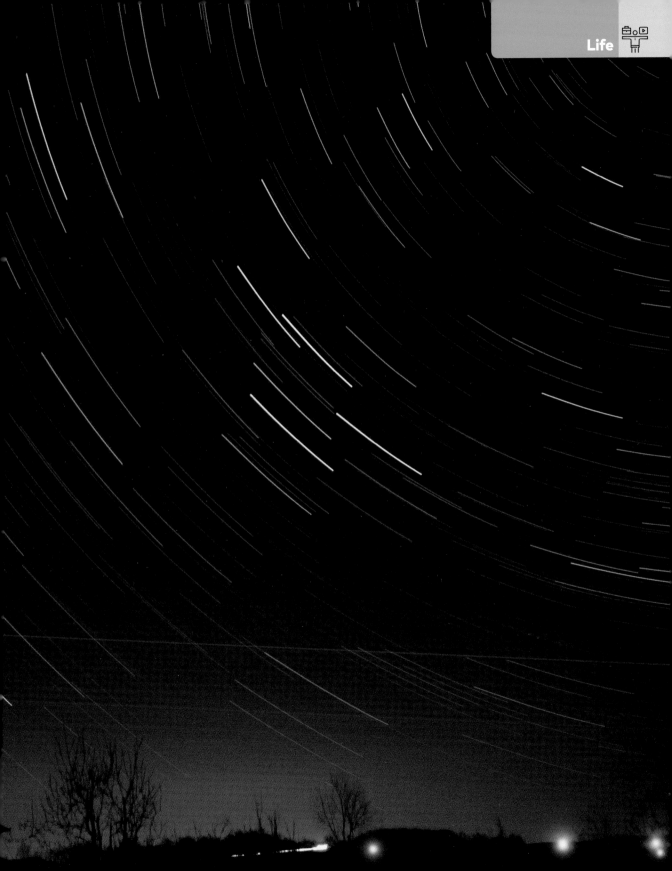

Why is sleep so important? The truth is we still don't have a fully comprehensive answer, but new research is constantly shining the light on some possible explanations. For instance, during the day metabolic "debris" accumulates between the connections in the brain and impairs the ability of nerve cells to communicate. When you sleep the gaps between brain cells open up and spinal fluid flows in, flushing out this junk. If you don't get enough good-quality sleep this process is limited. A recent online experiment that improved sleep among subjects was also successful at reducing depression, anxiety and paranoid thoughts.

7 ways to sleep better

Addressing any sleep issues and improving your sleep quality is one of the most important things you can do for better brain health and better overall health and happiness. Here's how you can sleep better tonight.

❶ Keep cool

A reduction in body temperature is a physiological indicator that it's nearly time for sleep. So if your room or bed is very hot, it makes it far harder to fall asleep and then stay asleep. Have the right tog duvet for the season and use a quiet fan if you need it. Taking a warm bath an hour before bed can also promote the onset of sleep because your body starts cooling down once you step out of the bath.

❷ Get some sun

Exposure to bright, natural light anchors your daily sleep/wake cycle in to a healthy rhythm. Try to get out and spend at least 30 minutes in daylight in the morning or take a half-hour walk after lunch.

❸ Hack your body clock

You may have heard of the circadian rhythm, which is the scientific name for your 24-hour body clock, but what about the ultradian rhythm? This is a 90-minute cycle that repeats throughout the day, and tracking yours can help you identify the best time for you to go to bed.

The ultradian rhythm is remarkably consistent and you can track it by timing your yawns. At the peak of the wave you're at your most alert and it's the perfect time to tackle your to-do list, but 45 minutes later you're at the trough of the wave and most likely to yawn. So, if you yawn around 8:30pm but it's too early to go to bed, you know you're likely to be most sleepy again at 10pm and then 11:30pm. You can then make sure you're in bed by 9:50pm or 11:20pm to get to sleep as quickly as possible.

❹ Put down your phone

Smartphones, tablets and computer screens emit blue light, which is the same wavelength as dawn light, and so is interpreted by your brain as a sign that it's take time wake up, be alert and get active. Try to avoid using your devices for at least an hour before bed or, at the very least, turn on your devices' night-time setting to shift from blue light to red light.

❺ Get blackout curtains

Make sure the room is as dark and quiet as possible and use an eye mask, blackout curtains and ear plugs if you live in or near a noisy environment. Remember that every bit of light or sound pollution can affect your ability to fall asleep and sleep soundly.

❻ Cut back on booze

Although alcohol promotes feelings of tiredness and can help you fall asleep, it disturbs your sleep quality by preventing your brain from entering the deeper, restorative phases of sleep. Try not to drink too much booze before going to bed, and cut back on all drinks: small-hours trips to the loo are very detrimental to a good night's sleep.

❼ Try to relax!

There is no magic number to how much sleep you need. The right amount is enough for you not to feel excessively sleepy during the day. That might be seven hours or nine; we all have different sleep needs. Work out how much you think you need then focus on getting that amount every night.

Quick tip

Good-quality sleep is essential to the health of your brain and body. The link between poor sleep and mood problems, weight gain, diabetes, severe depression and mental illness is clear. Put in the effort to improve your night-time routine and you should improve your physical health, energy, mood and well-being – not just this week or this month, but for years to come!

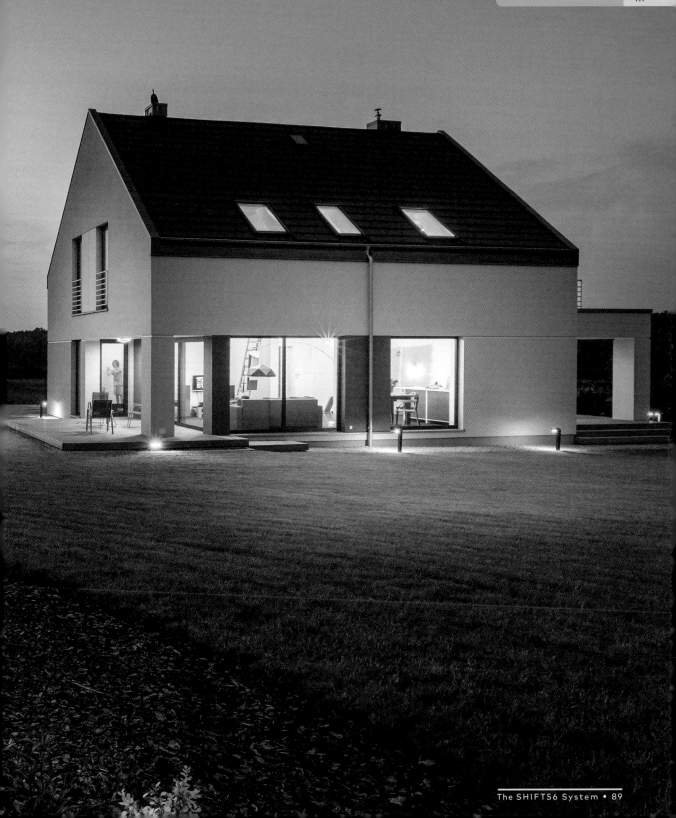

The SHIFT56 Journal

Here's why your new goal-setting journal is the key to a happier life!

It's probably been a while since you kept a journal or daily diary. It may have been a project set by your school or your parents over a school holiday (to keep you out of trouble!), or simply something you did for a while to record both the minor and major moments of your life.

But your journal is a very important part of The SHIFT56 System. It helps you to plan your day, note feelings, motivations, hopes and goals, and allows you to take a step back each day to appreciate the good things in your life. Journaling can also help you identify – and then overcome – any issues that are preventing you from being as happy as you want.

Journaling gives you complete control of your life, and empowers you to start making those small and sustainable habit changes that will allow you to realise all your hopes and ambitions and live the full, exciting and successful life you deserve. And we know it works: we've done it ourselves, and many high achievers in every arena from business to sport swear by it!

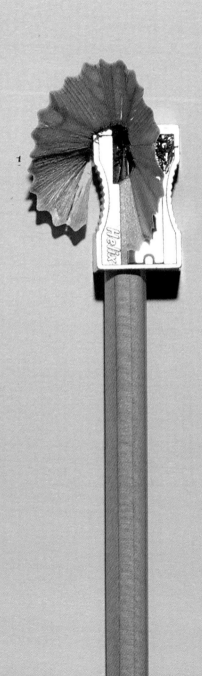

Train your brain!

In the next chapter you'll write down your number one health and happiness goal for the next eight weeks. We call this priority target your Big Picture Goal or BPG. We'll explain everything about setting your BPG, as well as your Weekly Achievable Goals or WAGs, on p104, but first here's how and why your journal will help you start living a healthier and happier life.

Journaling has a similar effect on your brain as exercising does on your body. Exercise makes your body fitter, stronger and leaner to enable you to move through life more easily, and journaling makes your brain better equipped to deal with the stresses and pressures life throws at you. And while your brain is an organ, it works like a muscle, so the more you do something the better you do it.

But keeping a journal, just like exercise, can be tricky at first. Opening a blank notebook, like entering a gym for the first time, can feel daunting and overwhelming. The good news is that in both scenarios the first time is always the hardest and you'll soon find it becomes much easier as you gain confidence and start to enjoy the experience.

So, just think of journaling like "training for your brain" to make your mind happier like exercise makes your body healthier. Yes, it takes practice but it quickly pays big rewards!

6 reasons you should start your journal

Journaling helps you take control of your life and become more positive, motivated and organised. There are many studies proving the life-changing benefits of journaling, and here are the top reasons you should start!

1 Journaling helps with the practice of mindfulness, calming your mind to allow you to focus on the present moment and reduce feelings of anxiety and stress and increase motivation and focus.

2 Being better connected to the present moment empowers you to identify, focus on and prioritise your goals, while managing negative emotions or feelings.

3 Becoming more self-aware and emotionally resilient allows you to quickly identify and deal with habits or factors stopping you from being happier.

4 The simple act of maintaining a daily journal increases self-discipline, which has crossover benefits in other areas of your life, such as work, eating and exercise.

5 It helps you think and communicate more clearly through a better understanding of your thoughts, feelings and emotions.

6 Writing something down – whether it's a thought or feeling, a to-do list, or the title of a book you've been recommended – is a powerful and permanent thing. Committing thoughts, reminders or ideas to paper prevents your brain from being overwhelmed by information so you can focus on important things.

What happens if I miss a day?
When life gets in the way it can be hard to make time, but busy periods are exactly when you need your journal to keep you on top of things! Have a plan B during hectic periods so you can keep your journal going. But if you do miss a day or two, don't worry! Just start again as soon as possible. It's like falling off your bike as a kid: the sooner you get back on the better, and the less likely you are to fall off again!

Journaling is a proven tool that will help improve your mood, motivation and mental well-being, increase your commitment to your goal, reduce your stress levels and enhance your quality of sleep, and much more besides! That's why we're convinced it's so worthwhile finding the time each day to do it. Turn the page to discover the quick and easy way to get started!

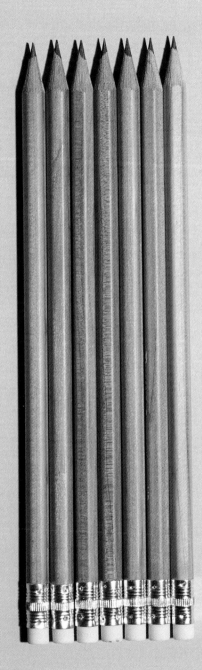

How to start your journal

Keeping your daily journal is one of the easiest steps towards a more exciting and fulfilling life!

Your daily journal is as important to your success on The SHIFT56 System as the exercise programme and eating guide. The three elements come together to multiply your health and happiness benefits by an even greater factor! Not only is your daily journal a great way to get on top of your day-to-day life, it's also a really important tool in helping you move quickly towards your number one health and happiness goal – your Big Picture Goal (BPG), which you'll set in the next chapter.

Before we explain how you can choose your BPG it's worth gaining a better understanding of how your journal works, in both providing immediate daily benefits and then keeping you on course to achieve your overall goal. Start your journal on the right foot and you will be amazed by how quickly you notice positive changes in every area of your life!

Is journaling difficult?
Keeping your own journal really couldn't be easier but, like when you start any new activity or habit, it can take a short period of adjustment before you feel fully at ease. Remember, the more often you do something the easier it becomes!

Does journaling take a lot of time and effort?
Can you spare two minutes in the morning and five minutes in the evening? That's all the time it takes to do your daily journal and change your life for the better! Once you start you'll realise these few minutes are among the most beneficial and helpful minutes of your day, and before long you won't believe how you managed without a journal before now.

I'm too busy to start a journal!
When you're stressed or busy it's tempting to think you don't have time to start or keep your journal. But it's during these more hectic times that journaling really comes into its own. It can prove invaluable in helping you get back on top of things so you don't have to feel overwhelmed again when life next gets challenging.

Your Daily Journal Explained
Here's how to bring your daily journal to life!

1 Day and Date
Make sure you write down today's day and date. It might seem obvious but it's another way to ensure you remain focused.

2 Morning
This part of your daily journal is done in the morning, ideally before you start your day.

3 Today's Word For The Day
This is your opportunity to think of one motivating or empowering word that you're going to keep in mind today – whatever happens! We recommend using words such as "strength", "positivity" or "focus" which we find keep us in the right frame of mind.

4 Today's Target
Rewrite the main goal you set last night that you want to achieve today.

5 Daily De-stresser
Write down the one thing or activity that you are going to do today that's just for you to help you relax, unwind and de-stress.

6 Evening
This part of your daily journal is done in the evening, ideally once you're back home after work or when you get into bed.

7 Big Win
Write down the one achievement today you're most proud of – and don't be modest or hold back: this is your opportunity to be loud and proud!

8 Lesson Learned
Write down the one main lesson you learned today that you are going to remember for the future.

9 Happy Highlight
Write down the one thing that happened today that made you laugh out loud or feel really happy and good about yourself and your life.

10 Tomorrow's Target
Write down the one thing that you would love to have achieved or completed by this time tomorrow.

11 Tonight's Thankfulness
Write down one thing that you feel thankful for today. It can be a big thing or a very small thing – that doesn't matter! It just needs to be something you're grateful for.

Journal
1 Day: ___
Date: __/__/__
2 Morning
3 Today's Word For The Day:
4 Today's Target — Today's number one priority I want to achieve is:
5 Daily De-stresser — My Daily De-stresser today will be:
6 Evening
7 Big Win — My Big Win today was:
Because:
8 Lesson Learned — Today I learned:
9 Happy Highlight — The highlight of my day was:
10 Tomorrow's Target — The one thing I want to have achieved by the end of the day tomorrow is:
11 Tonight's Thankfulness — Tonight I am thankful for:
Because:
108 - The SHIFT56 System

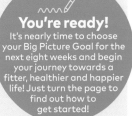
You're ready!
It's nearly time to choose your Big Picture Goal for the next eight weeks and begin your journey towards a fitter, healthier and happier life! Just turn the page to find out how to get started!

Overcoming obstacles

Here's how to keep your better-life journey progressing on the right track

In the next chapter you're going to set your Big Picture Goal or BPG – your number one health and happiness goal to work towards over the next eight weeks. Before you do, it's important to realise that there'll be some events or circumstances that could distract you from achieving your BPG. Some will be down to you (which we will call Internal Obstacles), some down to other people (External Obstacles), and others entirely outside your control (Uncontrollable Obstacles).

It doesn't matter what the obstacles are or where they originate. What matters is how you react to them so you can move past them quickly to get back on track. Having some strategies, which we call Positive Obstacle Plans (POPs), in mind will make overcoming them much easier!

The three types of obstacle
- An *Internal Obstacle* is a negative thought that questions your own ability to make positive changes to your life, or when you feel overwhelmed by how far you think you have to go to be healthier and happier.

- An *External Obstacle* is a negative thought or situation where we compare ourselves with other people, or where other people, for whatever reason, question your ability to make positive changes.

- An *Uncontrollable Obstacle* is a negative situation over which you have no control and can't really anticipate, such as you (or your kids) catching a cold, a last-minute work obligation or an injury.

Anticipating your obstacles
On a piece of paper write down three obstacles – one Internal, one External and one Uncontrollable – that could appear at some point over the next eight weeks, and then write down three (POPs) you will use if such an obstacle does arise (which, of course, there's every chance it won't!).

Here are three example obstacles to give you a better idea of what yours might be.

Internal Obstacle "I have failed to lose weight before and so I think I will fail again"
POP "I will remember that what has happened is in the past; what matters now is the future and I believe I am on the right path towards being healthier and happier for life"

External Obstacle "I will never be as lean or happy as that person"
POP "I will remember that I am unique and the only comparison I care about is whether I am healthier and happier than I was yesterday or last week. If I am, then I am doing everything right"

Uncontrollable Obstacle "I have caught a cold"
POP "I will remember that life is full of unexpected events – some good and some bad – but I will continue to follow my new daily healthy habits and fill in my daily journal until I feel well enough to exercise again"

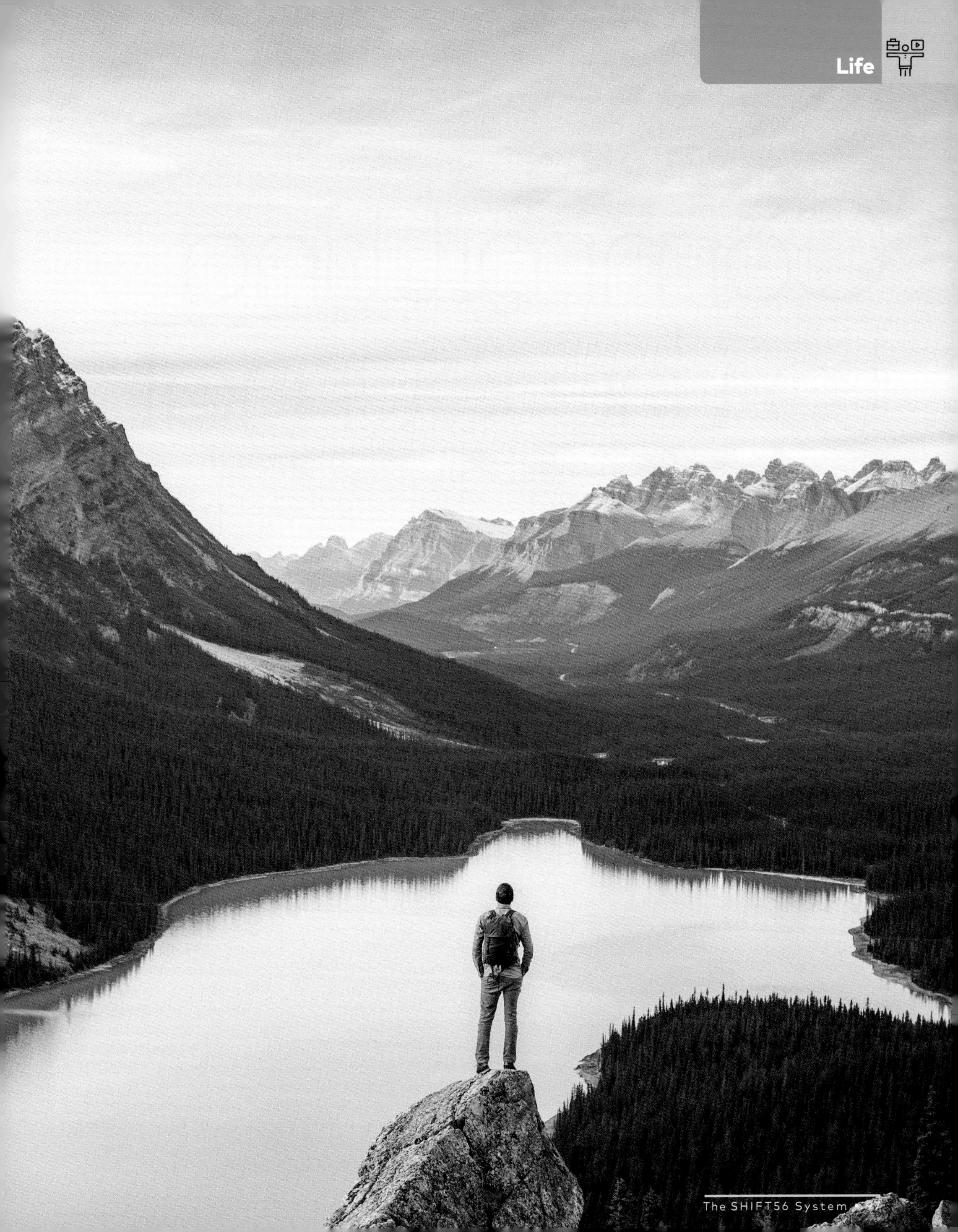

Committing to the journal

Make keeping your journal second nature and become happier than ever!

The easiest way to start your journal – and keep going – is to find some time that suits your regular routine. It may be as soon as you wake up or once you've eaten breakfast, or when you get in at the end of the day, or before getting into bed. It doesn't matter when you do your journal: doing it is more important! Here are three other ways to stay on track.

You're now ready to start your SHIFT56 Journal and start living a healthier and happier life!

❶ Keep it in sight

Journaling has the biggest positive benefits when it's done consistently, and you're more likely to do your journal if it's in sight and easy reach. Leaving it on your bedside table with a couple of pens will make your morning and evening entries easy to do, or you could even carry it in your work bag so you can journal when commuting or during some spare moments in the day.

❷ Ditch the distractions

Doing your daily journal entries doesn't take long, but you do need to be fully focused to get the greatest benefits. Move your phone and laptop away or turn off your notifications to give you some distraction-free time to fully engage with your journal. Doing it quickly and/or without your full attention won't deliver those big benefits you want.

❸ Talk about it

As well as improving your life, keeping a journal can help you have closer and deeper relationships with your friends and family, especially if they start their own journals too! Talking more about your thoughts, feelings, ambitions, fears and worries with people who care about you can help you focus on what you want out of life, and deal with challenges and difficulties.

Your Journal

Identifying your SHIFT56 goal

Here's how to choose your perfect goal to start living a healthier and happier life today!

You're reading The SHIFT56 System because you're determined to make big positive changes to the way you look and feel. And one of the most important first steps towards a healthier and happier life is to set a challenging yet realistic goal to work towards over the next eight weeks.

Identifying your number one health and fitness goal is both exciting and inspiring, but can also be a bit daunting. Don't worry – it's normal to feel a little worried about choosing the right goal! We're going to help you identify the best goal for you, and then what you need to do to make it a reality.

Your Big Picture Goal

Setting your priority goal, which we call your Big Picture Goal or BPG, requires you to think about what you can realistically achieve over the next eight weeks. Your BPG will be based on your unique circumstances, specifically your current health and fitness levels. We're all different, with different ideas of what a fitter, healthier and happier life means, so it's really important your BPG is tailored to you.

How do I choose my BPG?

Firstly, don't worry if you can't immediately think of a BPG. Here's a really good – and easy – exercise to help you find it. **In the big circle opposite write down all your main health and happiness goals – and don't be afraid to go big!** Think about those achievements that would make you really happy and proud of yourself if you made them a reality. Then go through your list and identify which are realistic within an eight-week timeframe. If you think some or all of them aren't possible within that time, simply tweak them to make them achievable. You now have a list of challenging but realistic goals!

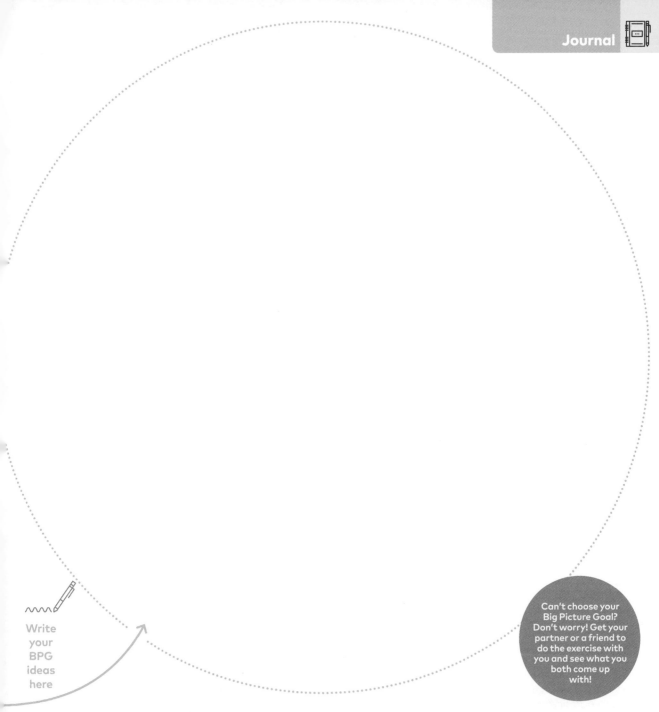

Write
your
BPG
ideas
here

Can't choose your
Big Picture Goal?
Don't worry! Get your
partner or a friend to
do the exercise with
you and see what you
both come up
with!

OK, now what do I do?

Now you must select your BPG from the list – the
one goal above all others you really want to achieve.
More often than not your BPG will jump off the
page! Again, don't worry if it feels a bit scary or
daunting. Once you start your BPG journey those
feelings will turn into excitement and motivation!

And don't discard your other goals – one of the
more challenging ones could end up being your *next*
BPG, while some of the smaller goals might form
your Weekly Achievable Goals (WAGs) to help you
achieve your BPG. Turn the page to find more about
your WAGs – and how to make your BPG a reality!

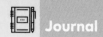

Making your Big Picture Goal a reality
Here's how your Weekly Achievable Goals help you hit your BPG!

What are my Weekly Achievable Goals?

Your Weekly Achievable Goals (WAGs) are mini-goals to achieve each week that will get you – and keep you – on track towards your BPG. Think of them like stepping stones to ensure you are progressing consistently towards your BPG, and give you little boosts of motivation and confidence along the way!

For example, let's look at someone whose BPG is to lose 12lb of fat in eight weeks.

Their Weekly Achievable Goals must complement their BPG, so some smart WAGs for Week 1 would be a fat loss target, an exercise target and an eating target.

Here's how this would appear in their journal:

My Week 1 WAGs to help me achieve my BPG are:

❶ **WAG 1**   Lose 1½lb of body fat

❷ **WAG 2**   Schedule my three weekly SHIFT56 workouts in my diary

❸ **WAG 3**   Do a weekly shop of delicious and nutritious food

Why are these smart WAGs?

WAG 1 is smart because... it breaks down your BPG into a much smaller and more achievable target. Losing body fat at a consistent rate is a much smarter way to get and then stay leaner.

WAG 2 is smart because... scheduling your weekly workouts like any other important appointment makes you far more likely to make time for exercise.

WAG 3 is smart because... filling your fridge and cupboards with more of the foods you know you need to eat means you're more likely to eat healthier more consistently!

What can I do each day to ensure I hit my Weekly Achievable Goals?

That's where your three Every Day Actions or EDAs come in! Quite simply, your EDAs are three really positive and easy new healthy habits you'll adopt each week to keep your progress moving in the right direction. Your three Week 1 EDAs need to be quite easy for you to put into action straight away. Then, as each week passes and you build more confidence and motivation, you can tweak or change your three EDAs each week to make them a little more challenging to improve your results!

Why are my WAGs and EDAs so important?

Having WAGs and EDAs makes you more accountable for your daily and weekly habits and actions that will help you achieve your BPG. Setting daily and weekly goals is a fantastic way to adopt healthy habits quickly and easily, and hitting these clear and simple targets will not only make you healthier and happier in their own right, but also make you realise – very quickly – how achievable your BPG is!

How do I select my three weekly EDAs?
It's really simple! Use these straightforward examples as inspiration

Here's what someone's Week 1 EDAs could be if their BPG is to lose 12lb of body fat in eight weeks.

WEEK 1
I will do the following three things every day this week to achieve my Week 1 WAGs

❶ **EDA 1**   I will drink 1.5 litres of water every day

❷ **EDA 2**   I will take a 20-minute walk before lunch, whatever the weather

❸ **EDA 3**   I will get up earlier and sit and eat breakfast at home before work

If that person successfully achieves all of these goals in Week 1 they may change or tweak some of their EDAs for Week 2, as follows...

WEEK 2
I will do the following three things every day this week to achieve my Week 2 WAGs

❶ **EDA 1**   I will drink 1.75l of water every day

❷ **EDA 2**   I will take a 30-minute walk after lunch, whatever the weather

❶ **EDA 3**   I will take my own home-made lunch to work every day

Whether you tweak your EDAs or change them completely, the most important thing is that each week you set three everyday goals you know you can achieve – even if they require a bit of thought, planning and effort!

Am I ready to get started on my BPG?

Almost! On the next page you'll write down your BPG. This includes why achieving it is so important to you, how it will improve your life – and how you'll reward yourself when you do!

Quick tip

Your Big Picture Goal (BPG) is your number one priority health and happiness goal that you want to (and will!) achieve in eight weeks.

Your Weekly Achievable Goals (WAGs) are three mini-goals that you'll set at the start of each week to keep you moving closer towards achieving your BPG.

Your Every Day Actions (EDAs) are three positive habits you'll set at the start of each week and then do daily to help you achieve that week's WAGs.

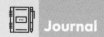

Setting your Big Picture Goal
Start living the life you've always wanted!

Over the previous pages you explored your desires and ambitions, and now you're ready to write down your Big Picture Goal and commit to it! Maybe it's something you've always wanted to make happen but never got around to putting the effort in. Or perhaps it's an entirely new goal that you identified by sitting down and making a list of your health and happiness ambitions.

If you still can't decide on your BPG, then don't worry: take a little time to relax and have a good think about what you really want out of life.

Once you've identified your BPG it's time to commit to it by writing it down on this page, along with the reasons this goal is so important to you, how achieving it would make you feel, and how you're going to reward yourself when you do!

Committing to your Big Picture Goal

Your BPG is your priority goal to focus on for the next eight weeks, and it's now time to write it down to start your journey towards achieving it!

My BPG is:

Achieving my BPG is very important to me because:

Achieving my BPG will make me feel:

Achieving my BPG will improve my life because:

Achieving my BPG means I will reward myself with:

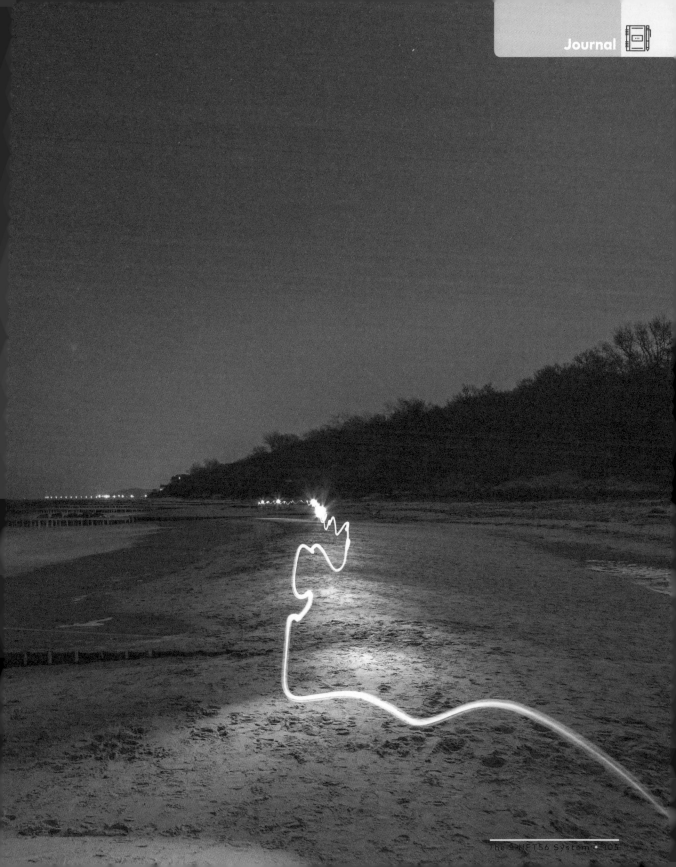

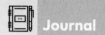

WEEK 1

My Weekly Achievable Goals (WAGs)
My WAGs for this week, to get me one week closer towards achieving my Big Picture Goal, are as follows:

❶ WAG 1:

❷ WAG 2:

❸ WAG 3:

Why are these WAGs so smart?
I have chosen these achievable WAGs for this week for the following reasons:

❶ WAG 1 is a smart weekly goal for me because:

❷ WAG 2 is a smart weekly goal for me because:

❸ WAG 3 is a smart weekly goal for me because:

WEEK 1

This week's Every Day Actions (EDAs)

I will do the following three things every day this week to help me achieve my Weekly Achievable Goals, which will help me achieve my Big Picture Goal:

❶ EDA 1:

❷ EDA 2:

❸ EDA 3:

Tracking my EDAs

	Mon	Tue	Wed	Thur	Fri	Sat	Sun	**Total**	**Goal hit?**
❶ EDA 1									
❷ EDA 2									
❸ EDA 3									

My week in five words

Here I choose five words that describe how achieving this week's WAGs and EDAs will make me feel:

Day: ....

Date: ..../........../...

Morning

Today's word for the day: ....

Today's Target
Today's number one priority I want to achieve is: ....

....

Daily De-stresser
My Daily De-stresser today will be: ....

....

Evening

Big Win
My Big Win today was: ....

....

Because: ....

....

Lesson Learned
Today I learned: ....

....

Happy Highlight
The highlight of my day was: ....

....

Tomorrow's Target
The one thing I want to have achieved by the end of the day tomorrow is: ....

....

Tonight's Thankfulness
Tonight I am thankful for: ....

....

Because: ....

....

Day: ....

Date: .... / .... / ....

Morning

Today's word for the day: ....

Today's Target
Today's number one priority I want to achieve is: ....

Daily De-stresser
My Daily De-stresser today will be: ....

Evening

Big Win
My Big Win today was: ....

Because: ....

Lesson Learned
Today I learned: ....

Happy Highlight
The highlight of my day was: ....

Tomorrow's Target
The one thing I want to have achieved by the end of the day tomorrow is: ...

Tonight's Thankfulness
Tonight I am thankful for: ....

Because: ....

Journal

Day: ....

Date: .... / .... / ....

Morning

Today's word for the day: ....

Today's Target
Today's number one priority I want to achieve is: ....

....

Daily De-stresser
My Daily De-stresser today will be: ....

....

Evening

Big Win
My Big Win today was: ....

....

Because: ....

....

Lesson Learned
Today I learned: ....

....

Happy Highlight
The highlight of my day was: ....

....

Tomorrow's Target
The one thing I want to have achieved by the end of the day tomorrow is: ....

....

Tonight's Thankfulness
Tonight I am thankful for: ....

....

Because: ....

....

Day: ....

Date: .... / .... / ....

Morning
Today's word for the day: ....

Today's Target
Today's number one priority I want to achieve is: ....

....

Daily De-stresser
My Daily De-stresser today will be: ....

....

Evening

Big Win
My Big Win today was: ....

....

Because: ....

....

Lesson Learned
Today I learned: ....

....

Happy Highlight
The highlight of my day was: ....

....

Tomorrow's Target
The one thing I want to have achieved by the end of the day tomorrow is: ....

....

Tonight's Thankfulness
Tonight I am thankful for: ....

....

Because: ....

....

Journal

Day: ....

Date: ..../......../...

Morning
Today's word for the day: ....

Today's Target
Today's number one priority I want to achieve is: ....

....

Daily De-stresser
My Daily De-stresser today will be: ....

....

Evening

Big Win
My Big Win today was: ....

....

Because: ....

....

Lesson Learned
Today I learned: ....

....

Happy Highlight
The highlight of my day was: ....

....

Tomorrow's Target
The one thing I want to have achieved by the end of the day tomorrow is: ....

....

Tonight's Thankfulness
Tonight I am thankful for: ....

....

Because: ....

....

Day: ....

Date: .... / .... / ....

Morning
Today's word for the day: ....

Today's Target
Today's number one priority I want to achieve is: ....

....

Daily De-stresser
My Daily De-stresser today will be: ....

....

Evening

Big Win
My Big Win today was: ....

....

Because: ....

....

Lesson Learned
Today I learned: ....

....

Happy Highlight
The highlight of my day was: ....

....

Tomorrow's Target
The one thing I want to have achieved by the end of the day tomorrow is: ....

....

Tonight's Thankfulness
Tonight I am thankful for: ....

....

Because: ....

....

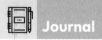

Journal

Day: ....

Date: .... / .... / ....

Morning

Today's word for the day: ....

Today's Target
Today's number one priority I want to achieve is: ....

....

Daily De-stresser
My Daily De-stresser today will be: ....

....

Evening

Big Win
My Big Win today was: ....

....

Because: ....

....

Lesson Learned
Today I learned: ....

....

Happy Highlight
The highlight of my day was: ....

....

Tomorrow's Target
The one thing I want to have achieved by the end of the day tomorrow is: ....

....

Tonight's Thankfulness
Tonight I am thankful for: ....

....

Because: ....

....

My Week In Review

Did I achieve my three WAGs? Circle the appropriate answer

❶ WAG 1:   Yes!   No   (If no, why not): ....

❷ WAG 2   Yes!   No   (If no, why not): ....

❸ WAG 3   Yes!   No   (If no, why not): ....

What was the best unexpected thing that happened to me this week, and why?

What things, if any, didn't go to plan this week?

What actions will I take to avoid this happening again?

What mark out of 10 do I give myself for the past week, and why?

Next week in focus
In a sentence, this is what I want to have achieved by the end of next week, and why:

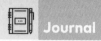
WEEK 2

My Weekly Achievable Goals (WAGs)

My WAGs for this week, to get me one week closer towards achieving my Big Picture Goal, are as follows:

❶ WAG 1:

❷ WAG 2:

❸ WAG 3:

Why are these WAGs so smart?

I have chosen these achievable WAGs for this week for the following reasons:

❶ WAG 1 is a smart weekly goal for me because:

❷ WAG 2 is a smart weekly goal for me because:

❸ WAG 3 is a smart weekly goal for me because:

WEEK 2

This week's Every Day Actions (EDAs)

I will do the following three things every day this week to help me achieve my Weekly Achievable Goals, which will help me achieve my Big Picture Goal:

❶ EDA 1:

❷ EDA 2:

❸ EDA 3:

Tracking my EDAs

	Mon	Tue	Wed	Thur	Fri	Sat	Sun	**Total**	**Goal hit?**
❶ EDA 1									
❷ EDA 2									
❸ EDA 3									

My week in five words

Here I choose five words that describe how achieving this week's WAGs and EDAs will make me feel:

Day: ....

Date: .... / .... / ....

Morning

Today's word for the day: ....

Today's Target
Today's number one priority I want to achieve is: ....
....

Daily De-stresser
My Daily De-stresser today will be: ....
....

Evening

Big Win
My Big Win today was: ....
....

Because: ....
....

Lesson Learned
Today I learned: ....
....

Happy Highlight
The highlight of my day was: ....
....

Tomorrow's Target
The one thing I want to have achieved by the end of the day tomorrow is: ....
....

Tonight's Thankfulness
Tonight I am thankful for: ....
....

Because: ....
....

Day: ....

Date: .... / .... / ....

Morning
Today's word for the day: ....

Today's Target
Today's number one priority I want to achieve is: ....
....

Daily De-stresser
My Daily De-stresser today will be: ....
....

Evening

Big Win
My Big Win today was: ....
....

Because: ....
....

Lesson Learned
Today I learned: ....
....

Happy Highlight
The highlight of my day was: ....
....

Tomorrow's Target
The one thing I want to have achieved by the end of the day tomorrow is: ....
....

Tonight's Thankfulness
Tonight I am thankful for: ....
....

Because: ....
....

Journal

Day: _____

Date: _____ / _____ / _____

Morning
Today's word for the day: _____

Today's Target
Today's number one priority I want to achieve is: _____

Daily De-stresser
My Daily De-stresser today will be: _____

Evening

Big Win
My Big Win today was: _____

Because: _____

Lesson Learned
Today I learned: _____

Happy Highlight
The highlight of my day was: _____

Tomorrow's Target
The one thing I want to have achieved by the end of the day tomorrow is: _____

Tonight's Thankfulness
Tonight I am thankful for: _____

Because: _____

Day: ....

Date: .... / .... / ....

Morning
Today's word for the day: ....

Today's Target
Today's number one priority I want to achieve is: ....

....

Daily De-stresser
My Daily De-stresser today will be: ....

....

Evening

Big Win
My Big Win today was: ....

....

Because: ....

....

Lesson Learned
Today I learned: ....

....

Happy Highlight
The highlight of my day was: ....

....

Tomorrow's Target
The one thing I want to have achieved by the end of the day tomorrow is: ....

....

Tonight's Thankfulness
Tonight I am thankful for: ....

....

Because: ....

....

Journal

Day: ....

Date: ..../......../...

Morning

Today's word for the day: ....

Today's Target
Today's number one priority I want to achieve is: ....
....

Daily De-stresser
My Daily De-stresser today will be: ....
....

Evening

Big Win
My Big Win today was: ....
....

Because: ....
....

Lesson Learned
Today I learned: ....
....

Happy Highlight
The highlight of my day was: ....
....

Tomorrow's Target
The one thing I want to have achieved by the end of the day tomorrow is: ....
....

Tonight's Thankfulness
Tonight I am thankful for: ....
....

Because: ....
....

Day: ....

Date: ..../......../........

Morning

Today's word for the day: ....

Today's Target
Today's number one priority I want to achieve is: ....
....

Daily De-stresser
My Daily De-stresser today will be: ....
....

Evening

Big Win
My Big Win today was: ....
....

Because: ....
....

Lesson Learned
Today I learned: ....
....

Happy Highlight
The highlight of my day was: ....
....

Tomorrow's Target
The one thing I want to have achieved by the end of the day tomorrow is: ....
....

Tonight's Thankfulness
Tonight I am thankful for: ....
....

Because: ....
....

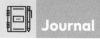

Journal

Day: ....

Date: .... / .... / ....

Morning

Today's word for the day: ....

Today's Target
Today's number one priority I want to achieve is: ....

....

Daily De-stresser
My Daily De-stresser today will be: ....

....

Evening

Big Win
My Big Win today was: ....

....

Because: ....

....

Lesson Learned
Today I learned: ....

....

Happy Highlight
The highlight of my day was: ....

....

Tomorrow's Target
The one thing I want to have achieved by the end of the day tomorrow is: ....

....

Tonight's Thankfulness
Tonight I am thankful for: ....

....

Because: ....

....

My Week In Review

Did I achieve my three WAGs? Circle the appropriate answer

❶ WAG 1:   Yes!   No   (If no, why not): ....

❷ WAG 2   Yes!   No   (If no, why not): ....

❸ WAG 3   Yes!   No   (If no, why not): ....

What was the best unexpected thing that happened to me this week, and why?

....

....

What things, if any, didn't go to plan this week?

....

....

What actions will I take to avoid this happening again?

....

....

What mark out of 10 do I give myself for the past week, and why?

....

....

Next week in focus
In a sentence, this is what I want to have achieved by the end of next week, and why:

....

....

....

....

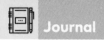

WEEK 3

My Weekly Achievable Goals (WAGs)

My WAGs for this week, to get me one week closer towards achieving my Big Picture Goal, are as follows:

❶ WAG 1:

❷ WAG 2:

❸ WAG 3:

Why are these WAGs so smart?

I have chosen these achievable WAGs for this week for the following reasons:

❶ WAG 1 is a smart weekly goal for me because:

❷ WAG 2 is a smart weekly goal for me because:

❸ WAG 3 is a smart weekly goal for me because:

WEEK 3

This week's Every Day Actions (EDAs)

I will do the following three things every day this week to help me achieve my Weekly Achievable Goals, which will help me achieve my Big Picture Goal:

❶ EDA 1:

❷ EDA 2:

❸ EDA 3:

Tracking my EDAs

	Mon	Tue	Wed	Thur	Fri	Sat	Sun	**Total**	**Goal hit?**
❶ EDA 1									
❷ EDA 2									
❸ EDA 3									

My week in five words

Here I choose five words that describe how achieving this week's WAGs and EDAs will make me feel:

Journal

Day: ....

Date: .... / .... / ....

Morning
Today's word for the day: ....

Today's Target
Today's number one priority I want to achieve is: ....

....

Daily De-stresser
My Daily De-stresser today will be: ....

....

Evening

Big Win
My Big Win today was: ....

....

Because: ....

....

Lesson Learned
Today I learned: ....

....

Happy Highlight
The highlight of my day was: ....

....

Tomorrow's Target
The one thing I want to have achieved by the end of the day tomorrow is: ....

....

Tonight's Thankfulness
Tonight I am thankful for: ....

....

Because: ....

....

Day: ....

Date: .... / .... / ....

Morning
Today's word for the day: ....

Today's Target
Today's number one priority I want to achieve is: ....
....

Daily De-stresser
My Daily De-stresser today will be: ....
....

Evening

Big Win
My Big Win today was: ....
....

Because: ....
....

Lesson Learned
Today I learned: ....
....

Happy Highlight
The highlight of my day was: ....
....

Tomorrow's Target
The one thing I want to have achieved by the end of the day tomorrow is: ....
....

Tonight's Thankfulness
Tonight I am thankful for: ....
....

Because: ....
....

Journal

Day: ....

Date: .... / .... / ....

Morning

Today's word for the day: ....

Today's Target
Today's number one priority I want to achieve is: ....
....

Daily De-stresser
My Daily De-stresser today will be: ....
....

Evening

Big Win
My Big Win today was: ....
....

Because: ....
....

Lesson Learned
Today I learned: ....
....

Happy Highlight
The highlight of my day was: ....
....

Tomorrow's Target
The one thing I want to have achieved by the end of the day tomorrow is: ....
....

Tonight's Thankfulness
Tonight I am thankful for: ....
....

Because: ....
....

Day: ....

Date: .... / .... / ....

Morning
Today's word for the day: ....

Today's Target
Today's number one priority I want to achieve is: ....

....

Daily De-stresser
My Daily De-stresser today will be: ....

....

Evening

Big Win
My Big Win today was: ....

....

Because: ....

....

Lesson Learned
Today I learned: ....

....

Happy Highlight
The highlight of my day was: ....

....

Tomorrow's Target
The one thing I want to have achieved by the end of the day tomorrow is: ....

....

Tonight's Thankfulness
Tonight I am thankful for: ....

....

Because: ....

....

Day: ....

Date: .... / .... / ....

Morning

Today's word for the day: ....

Today's Target
Today's number one priority I want to achieve is: ....
....

Daily De-stresser
My Daily De-stresser today will be: ....
....

Evening

Big Win
My Big Win today was: ....
....

Because: ....
....

Lesson Learned
Today I learned: ....
....

Happy Highlight
The highlight of my day was: ....
....

Tomorrow's Target
The one thing I want to have achieved by the end of the day tomorrow is: ....
....

Tonight's Thankfulness
Tonight I am thankful for: ....
....

Because: ....
....

Day: ....

Date: .... / .... / ....

Morning
Today's word for the day: ....

Today's Target
Today's number one priority I want to achieve is: ....
....

Daily De-stresser
My Daily De-stresser today will be: ....
....

Evening

Big Win
My Big Win today was: ....
....

Because: ....
....

Lesson Learned
Today I learned: ....
....

Happy Highlight
The highlight of my day was: ....
....

Tomorrow's Target
The one thing I want to have achieved by the end of the day tomorrow is: ....
....

Tonight's Thankfulness
Tonight I am thankful for: ....
....

Because: ....
....

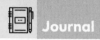

Day: ....

Date: ..../........../...

Morning

Today's word for the day: ....

Today's Target
Today's number one priority I want to achieve is: ....

....

Daily De-stresser
My Daily De-stresser today will be: ....

....

Evening

Big Win
My Big Win today was: ....

....

Because: ....

....

Lesson Learned
Today I learned: ....

....

Happy Highlight
The highlight of my day was: ....

....

Tomorrow's Target
The one thing I want to have achieved by the end of the day tomorrow is: ....

....

Tonight's Thankfulness
Tonight I am thankful for: ....

....

Because: ....

....

My Week In Review

Did I achieve my three WAGs? Circle the appropriate answer

❶ WAG 1:   Yes!   No   (If no, why not): ....

❷ WAG 2   Yes!   No   (If no, why not): ....

❸ WAG 3   Yes!   No   (If no, why not): ....

What was the best unexpected thing that happened to me this week, and why?

....

....

What things, if any, didn't go to plan this week?

....

....

What actions will I take to avoid this happening again?

....

....

What mark out of 10 do I give myself for the past week, and why?

....

....

Next week in focus
In a sentence, this is what I want to have achieved by the end of next week, and why:

....

....

....

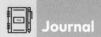

My Weekly Achievable Goals (WAGs)

My WAGs for this week, to get me one week closer towards achieving my Big Picture Goal, are as follows:

❶ WAG 1: ....

....

❷ WAG 2: ....

....

❸ WAG 3: ....

....

....

Why are these WAGs so smart?

I have chosen these achievable WAGs for this week for the following reasons:

❶ WAG 1 is a smart weekly goal for me because: ....

....

....

....

❷ WAG 2 is a smart weekly goal for me because: ....

....

....

....

❸ WAG 3 is a smart weekly goal for me because: ....

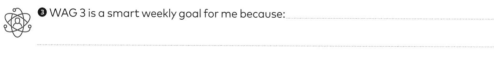

....

....

....

This week's Every Day Actions (EDAs)

I will do the following three things every day this week to help me achieve my Weekly Achievable Goals, which will help me achieve my Big Picture Goal:

❶ EDA 1:

❷ EDA 2:

❸ EDA 3:

Tracking my EDAs

	Mon	Tue	Wed	Thur	Fri	Sat	Sun	Total	Goal hit?
❶ EDA 1									
❷ EDA 2									
❸ EDA 3									

My week in five words

Here I choose five words that describe how achieving this week's WAGs and EDAs will make me feel:

Day: ....

Date: ..../......../........

Morning

Today's word for the day: ....

Today's Target
Today's number one priority I want to achieve is: ....

....

Daily De-stresser
My Daily De-stresser today will be: ....

....

Evening

Big Win
My Big Win today was: ....

....

Because: ....

....

Lesson Learned
Today I learned: ....

....

Happy Highlight
The highlight of my day was: ....

....

Tomorrow's Target
The one thing I want to have achieved by the end of the day tomorrow is: ....

....

Tonight's Thankfulness
Tonight I am thankful for: ....

....

Because: ....

....

Day: ....

Date: .... / .... / ....

Morning
Today's word for the day: ....

Today's Target
Today's number one priority I want to achieve is: ....

....

Daily De-stresser
My Daily De-stresser today will be: ....

....

Evening

Big Win
My Big Win today was: ....

....

Because: ....

....

Lesson Learned
Today I learned: ....

....

Happy Highlight
The highlight of my day was: ....

....

Tomorrow's Target
The one thing I want to have achieved by the end of the day tomorrow is: ....

....

Tonight's Thankfulness
Tonight I am thankful for: ....

....

Because: ....

....

Journal

Day: ....

Date: .... / .... / ....

Morning
Today's word for the day: ....

Today's Target
Today's number one priority I want to achieve is: ....

....

Daily De-stresser
My Daily De-stresser today will be: ....

....

Evening

Big Win
My Big Win today was: ....

....

Because: ....

....

Lesson Learned
Today I learned: ....

....

Happy Highlight
The highlight of my day was: ....

....

Tomorrow's Target
The one thing I want to have achieved by the end of the day tomorrow is: ....

....

Tonight's Thankfulness
Tonight I am thankful for: ....

....

Because: ....

....

Day: ....

Date: .... / .... / ....

Morning
Today's word for the day: ....

Today's Target
Today's number one priority I want to achieve is: ....
....

Daily De-stresser
My Daily De-stresser today will be: ....
....

Evening

Big Win
My Big Win today was: ....
....

Because: ....
....

Lesson Learned
Today I learned: ....
....

Happy Highlight
The highlight of my day was: ....
....

Tomorrow's Target
The one thing I want to have achieved by the end of the day tomorrow is: ....
....

Tonight's Thankfulness
Tonight I am thankful for: ....
....

Because: ....
....

Day: ....

Date: .... / .... / ....

Morning
Today's word for the day: ....

Today's Target
Today's number one priority I want to achieve is: ....

....

Daily De-stresser
My Daily De-stresser today will be: ....

....

Evening

Big Win
My Big Win today was: ....

....

Because: ....

....

Lesson Learned
Today I learned: ....

....

Happy Highlight
The highlight of my day was: ....

....

Tomorrow's Target
The one thing I want to have achieved by the end of the day tomorrow is: ....

....

Tonight's Thankfulness
Tonight I am thankful for: ....

....

Because: ....

....

Day: _____

Date: ____ / ____ / ____

Morning

Today's word for the day: _____

Today's Target
Today's number one priority I want to achieve is: _____

Daily De-stresser
My Daily De-stresser today will be: _____

Evening

Big Win
My Big Win today was: _____

Because: _____

Lesson Learned
Today I learned: _____

Happy Highlight
The highlight of my day was: _____

Tomorrow's Target
The one thing I want to have achieved by the end of the day tomorrow is: _____

Tonight's Thankfulness
Tonight I am thankful for: _____

Because: _____

Day: ....

Date: .... / .... / ....

Morning

Today's word for the day: ....

Today's Target
Today's number one priority I want to achieve is: ....
....

Daily De-stresser
My Daily De-stresser today will be: ....
....

Evening

Big Win
My Big Win today was: ....
....

Because: ....
....

Lesson Learned
Today I learned: ....
....

Happy Highlight
The highlight of my day was: ....
....

Tomorrow's Target
The one thing I want to have achieved by the end of the day tomorrow is: ....
....

Tonight's Thankfulness
Tonight I am thankful for: ....
....

Because: ....
....

My Week In Review

Did I achieve my three WAGs? Circle the appropriate answer

❶ WAG 1:   Yes!   No   (If no, why not): ....

❷ WAG 2   Yes!   No   (If no, why not): ....

❸ WAG 3   Yes!   No   (If no, why not): ....

What was the best unexpected thing that happened to me this week, and why?

....

....

What things, if any, didn't go to plan this week?

....

....

....

What actions will I take to avoid this happening again?

....

....

....

What mark out of 10 do I give myself for the past week, and why?

....

....

....

Next week in focus
In a sentence, this is what I want to have achieved by the end of next week, and why:

....

....

....

....

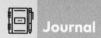
WEEK 5

My Weekly Achievable Goals (WAGs)

My WAGs for this week, to get me one week closer towards achieving my Big Picture Goal, are as follows:

❶ WAG 1: ....

❷ WAG 2: ....

❸ WAG 3: ....

Why are these WAGs so smart?

I have chosen these achievable WAGs for this week for the following reasons:

❶ WAG 1 is a smart weekly goal for me because: ....

❷ WAG 2 is a smart weekly goal for me because: ....

❸ WAG 3 is a smart weekly goal for me because: ....

WEEK 5

This week's Every Day Actions (EDAs)

I will do the following three things every day this week to help me achieve my Weekly Achievable Goals, which will help me achieve my Big Picture Goal:

❶ EDA 1:

❷ EDA 2:

❸ EDA 3:

Tracking my EDAs

	Mon	Tue	Wed	Thur	Fri	Sat	Sun	**Total**	**Goal hit?**
❶ EDA 1									
❷ EDA 2									
❸ EDA 3									

My week in five words

Here I choose five words that describe how achieving this week's WAGs and EDAs will make me feel:

Journal

Day: ....

Date: .... / .... / ....

Morning
Today's word for the day: ....

Today's Target
Today's number one priority I want to achieve is: ....
....

Daily De-stresser
My Daily De-stresser today will be: ....
....

Evening

Big Win
My Big Win today was: ....
....

Because: ....
....

Lesson Learned
Today I learned: ....
....

Happy Highlight
The highlight of my day was: ....
....

Tomorrow's Target
The one thing I want to have achieved by the end of the day tomorrow is: ....
....

Tonight's Thankfulness
Tonight I am thankful for: ....
....

Because: ....
....

Day: ....

Date: ..../............/............

Morning

Today's word for the day: ....

Today's Target
Today's number one priority I want to achieve is: ....

Daily De-stresser
My Daily De-stresser today will be: ....
....

Evening

Big Win
My Big Win today was: ....
....

Because: ....
....

Lesson Learned
Today I learned: ....
....

Happy Highlight
The highlight of my day was: ....
....

Tomorrow's Target
The one thing I want to have achieved by the end of the day tomorrow is: ....
....

Tonight's Thankfulness
Tonight I am thankful for: ....
....

Because: ....
....

Journal

Day: ....

Date: .... / .... / ....

Morning
Today's word for the day: ....

Today's Target
Today's number one priority I want to achieve is: ....

....

Daily De-stresser
My Daily De-stresser today will be: ....

....

Evening

Big Win
My Big Win today was: ....

....

Because: ....

....

Lesson Learned
Today I learned: ....

....

Happy Highlight
The highlight of my day was: ....

....

Tomorrow's Target
The one thing I want to have achieved by the end of the day tomorrow is: ....

....

Tonight's Thankfulness
Tonight I am thankful for: ....

....

Because: ....

....

Day:

Date: _____ / _____ / _____

Morning

Today's word for the day:

Today's Target
Today's number one priority I want to achieve is:

Daily De-stresser
My Daily De-stresser today will be:

Evening

Big Win
My Big Win today was:

Because:

Lesson Learned
Today I learned:

Happy Highlight
The highlight of my day was:

Tomorrow's Target
The one thing I want to have achieved by the end of the day tomorrow is:

Tonight's Thankfulness
Tonight I am thankful for:

Because:

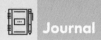
Journal

Day: ....

Date: .... / .... / ....

Morning
Today's word for the day: ....

Today's Target
Today's number one priority I want to achieve is: ....
....

Daily De-stresser
My Daily De-stresser today will be: ....
....

Evening

Big Win
My Big Win today was: ....
....

Because: ....
....

Lesson Learned
Today I learned: ....
....

Happy Highlight
The highlight of my day was: ....
....

Tomorrow's Target
The one thing I want to have achieved by the end of the day tomorrow is: ....
....

Tonight's Thankfulness
Tonight I am thankful for: ....
....

Because: ....
....

Day: ....

Date: .... / .... / ....

Morning

Today's word for the day: ....

Today's Target
Today's number one priority I want to achieve is: ....
....

Daily De-stresser
My Daily De-stresser today will be: ....
....

Evening

Big Win
My Big Win today was: ....
....

Because: ....
....

Lesson Learned
Today I learned: ....
....

Happy Highlight
The highlight of my day was: ....
....

Tomorrow's Target
The one thing I want to have achieved by the end of the day tomorrow is: ....
....

Tonight's Thankfulness
Tonight I am thankful for: ....
....

Because: ....
....

Journal

Day: ....

Date: .... / .... / ....

Morning

Today's word for the day: ....

Today's Target
Today's number one priority I want to achieve is: ....
....

Daily De-stresser
My Daily De-stresser today will be: ....
....

Evening

Big Win
My Big Win today was: ....
....

Because: ....
....

Lesson Learned
Today I learned: ....
....

Happy Highlight
The highlight of my day was: ....
....

Tomorrow's Target
The one thing I want to have achieved by the end of the day tomorrow is: ....
....

Tonight's Thankfulness
Tonight I am thankful for: ....
....

Because: ....
....

My Week In Review

Did I achieve my three WAGs? Circle the appropriate answer

❶ WAG 1:   Yes!   No   (If no, why not): ....
....

❷ WAG 2   Yes!   No   (If no, why not): ....
....

❸ WAG 3   Yes!   No   (If no, why not): ....
....

What was the best unexpected thing that happened to me this week, and why?
....
....

What things, if any, didn't go to plan this week?
....
....

What actions will I take to avoid this happening again?
....
....

What mark out of 10 do I give myself for the past week, and why?
....
....

Next week in focus
In a sentence, this is what I want to have achieved by the end of next week, and why:
....
....
....

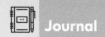

My Weekly Achievable Goals (WAGs)

My WAGs for this week, to get me one week closer towards achieving my Big Picture Goal, are as follows:

❶ WAG 1:

❷ WAG 2:

❸ WAG 3:

Why are these WAGs so smart?

I have chosen these achievable WAGs for this week for the following reasons:

❶ WAG 1 is a smart weekly goal for me because:

❷ WAG 2 is a smart weekly goal for me because:

❸ WAG 3 is a smart weekly goal for me because:

WEEK 6

This week's Every Day Actions (EDAs)

I will do the following three things every day this week to help me achieve my Weekly Achievable Goals, which will help me achieve my Big Picture Goal:

❶ EDA 1: ....
....

❷ EDA 2: ....
....

❸ EDA 3: ....
....

Tracking my EDAs

	Mon	Tue	Wed	Thur	Fri	Sat	Sun	**Total**	**Goal hit?**
❶ EDA 1									
❷ EDA 2									
❸ EDA 3									

My week in five words

Here I choose five words that describe how achieving this week's WAGs and EDAs will make me feel:

✓ ....

✓ ....

✓ ....

✓ ....

✓ ....

Journal

Day: ....

Date: ..../......../........

Morning
Today's word for the day: ....

Today's Target
Today's number one priority I want to achieve is: ....
....

Daily De-stresser
My Daily De-stresser today will be: ....
....

Evening

Big Win
My Big Win today was: ....
....

Because: ....
....

Lesson Learned
Today I learned: ....
....

Happy Highlight
The highlight of my day was: ....
....

Tomorrow's Target
The one thing I want to have achieved by the end of the day tomorrow is: ....
....

Tonight's Thankfulness
Tonight I am thankful for: ....
....

Because: ....
....

Day: ....

Date: .... / .... / ....

Morning

Today's word for the day: ....

Today's Target
Today's number one priority I want to achieve is: ....
....

Daily De-stresser
My Daily De-stresser today will be: ....
....

Evening

Big Win
My Big Win today was: ....
....

Because: ....
....

Lesson Learned
Today I learned: ....
....

Happy Highlight
The highlight of my day was: ....
....

Tomorrow's Target
The one thing I want to have achieved by the end of the day tomorrow is: ....
....

Tonight's Thankfulness
Tonight I am thankful for: ....
....

Because: ....
....

Journal

Day: ....

Date: ..../......../........

Morning
Today's word for the day: ....

Today's Target
Today's number one priority I want to achieve is: ....
....

Daily De-stresser
My Daily De-stresser today will be: ....
....

Evening

Big Win
My Big Win today was: ....

Because: ....

Lesson Learned
Today I learned: ....

Happy Highlight
The highlight of my day was: ....

Tomorrow's Target
The one thing I want to have achieved by the end of the day tomorrow is: ....

Tonight's Thankfulness
Tonight I am thankful for: ....

Because: ....

Day: ....

Date: .... / .... / ....

Morning

Today's word for the day: ....

Today's Target
Today's number one priority I want to achieve is: ....
....

Daily De-stresser
My Daily De-stresser today will be: ....
....

Evening

Big Win
My Big Win today was: ....
....

Because: ....
....

Lesson Learned
Today I learned: ....
....

Happy Highlight
The highlight of my day was: ....
....

Tomorrow's Target
The one thing I want to have achieved by the end of the day tomorrow is: ....
....

Tonight's Thankfulness
Tonight I am thankful for: ....
....

Because: ....
....

Journal

Day: ....

Date: .... / .... / ....

Morning

Today's word for the day: ....

Today's Target
Today's number one priority I want to achieve is: ....

....

Daily De-stresser
My Daily De-stresser today will be: ....

....

Evening

Big Win
My Big Win today was: ....

....

Because: ....

....

Lesson Learned
Today I learned: ....

....

Happy Highlight
The highlight of my day was: ....

....

Tomorrow's Target
The one thing I want to have achieved by the end of the day tomorrow is: ......

....

Tonight's Thankfulness
Tonight I am thankful for: ....

....

Because: ....

....

Day: ....

Date: .... / .... / ....

Morning

Today's word for the day: ....

Today's Target
Today's number one priority I want to achieve is: ....
....

Daily De-stresser
My Daily De-stresser today will be: ....
....

Evening

Big Win
My Big Win today was: ....
....

Because: ....
....

Lesson Learned
Today I learned: ....
....

Happy Highlight
The highlight of my day was: ....
....

Tomorrow's Target
The one thing I want to have achieved by the end of the day tomorrow is: ....
....

Tonight's Thankfulness
Tonight I am thankful for: ....
....

Because: ....
....

Day: ....

Date: .... / .... / ....

Morning
Today's word for the day: ....

Today's Target
Today's number one priority I want to achieve is: ....
....

Daily De-stresser
My Daily De-stresser today will be: ....
....

Evening

Big Win
My Big Win today was: ....
....

Because: ....
....

Lesson Learned
Today I learned: ....
....

Happy Highlight
The highlight of my day was: ....
....

Tomorrow's Target
The one thing I want to have achieved by the end of the day tomorrow is: ....
....

Tonight's Thankfulness
Tonight I am thankful for: ....
....

Because: ....
....

My Week In Review

Did I achieve my three WAGs? Circle the appropriate answer

❶ WAG 1:   Yes!   No   (If no, why not): ....

❷ WAG 2   Yes!   No   (If no, why not): ....

❸ WAG 3   Yes!   No   (If no, why not): ....

What was the best unexpected thing that happened to me this week, and why?

....

....

What things, if any, didn't go to plan this week?

....

....

What actions will I take to avoid this happening again?

....

....

What mark out of 10 do I give myself for the past week, and why?

....

....

Next week in focus
In a sentence, this is what I want to have achieved by the end of next week, and why:

....

....

....

....

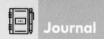

WEEK 7

My Weekly Achievable Goals (WAGs)

My WAGs for this week, to get me one week closer towards achieving my Big Picture Goal, are as follows:

❶ WAG 1:

❷ WAG 2:

❸ WAG 3:

Why are these WAGs so smart?

I have chosen these achievable WAGs for this week for the following reasons:

❶ WAG 1 is a smart weekly goal for me because:

❷ WAG 2 is a smart weekly goal for me because:

❸ WAG 3 is a smart weekly goal for me because:

WEEK 7

This week's Every Day Actions (EDAs)

I will do the following three things every day this week to help me achieve my Weekly Achievable Goals, which will help me achieve my Big Picture Goal:

❶ EDA 1: ....

....

....

❷ EDA 2: ....

....

....

❸ EDA 3: ....

....

....

Tracking my EDAs

	Mon	Tue	Wed	Thur	Fri	Sat	Sun	**Total**	**Goal hit?**
❶ EDA 1									
❷ EDA 2									
❸ EDA 3									

My week in five words

Here I choose five words that describe how achieving this week's WAGs and EDAs will make me feel:

⊘ ....

⊘ ....

⊘ ....

⊘ ....

⊘ ....

Day: ....

Date: .... / .... / ....

Morning

Today's word for the day: ....

🎯 Today's Target
Today's number one priority I want to achieve is: ....

....

🧘 Daily De-stresser
My Daily De-stresser today will be: ....

....

Evening

🏆 Big Win
My Big Win today was: ....

....

Because: ....

....

🧲 Lesson Learned
Today I learned: ....

....

🙆 Happy Highlight
The highlight of my day was: ....

....

🎯 Tomorrow's Target
The one thing I want to have achieved by the end of the day tomorrow is: ....

....

🌱 Tonight's Thankfulness
Tonight I am thankful for: ....

....

Because: ....

....

Day: ....

Date: ..../......../........

Morning

Today's word for the day: ....

Today's Target
Today's number one priority I want to achieve is: ....

....

Daily De-stresser
My Daily De-stresser today will be: ....

....

Evening

Big Win
My Big Win today was: ....

....

Because: ....

....

Lesson Learned
Today I learned: ....

....

Happy Highlight
The highlight of my day was: ....

....

Tomorrow's Target
The one thing I want to have achieved by the end of the day tomorrow is: ....

....

Tonight's Thankfulness
Tonight I am thankful for: ....

....

Because: ....

....

Journal

Day: ....

Date: .... / .... / ....

Morning
Today's word for the day: ....

Today's Target
Today's number one priority I want to achieve is: ....
....

Daily De-stresser
My Daily De-stresser today will be: ....
....

Evening

Big Win
My Big Win today was: ....
....

Because: ....
....

Lesson Learned
Today I learned: ....
....

Happy Highlight
The highlight of my day was: ....
....

Tomorrow's Target
The one thing I want to have achieved by the end of the day tomorrow is: ....
....

Tonight's Thankfulness
Tonight I am thankful for: ....
....

Because: ....
....

Day:

Date: ___ / ___ / ___

Morning

Today's word for the day:

Today's Target
Today's number one priority I want to achieve is:

Daily De-stresser
My Daily De-stresser today will be:

Evening

Big Win
My Big Win today was:

Because:

Lesson Learned
Today I learned:

Happy Highlight
The highlight of my day was:

Tomorrow's Target
The one thing I want to have achieved by the end of the day tomorrow is:

Tonight's Thankfulness
Tonight I am thankful for:

Because:

Day: ....

Date: .... / .... / ....

Morning

Today's word for the day: ....

Today's Target
Today's number one priority I want to achieve is: ....

....

Daily De-stresser
My Daily De-stresser today will be: ....

....

Evening

Big Win
My Big Win today was: ....

....

Because: ....

....

Lesson Learned
Today I learned: ....

....

Happy Highlight
The highlight of my day was: ....

....

Tomorrow's Target
The one thing I want to have achieved by the end of the day tomorrow is: ....

....

Tonight's Thankfulness
Tonight I am thankful for: ....

....

Because: ....

....

Day: ....

Date: .... / .... / ....

Morning

Today's word for the day: ....

Today's Target
Today's number one priority I want to achieve is: ....

....

Daily De-stresser
My Daily De-stresser today will be: ....

....

Evening

Big Win
My Big Win today was: ....

....

Because: ....

....

Lesson Learned
Today I learned: ....

....

Happy Highlight
The highlight of my day was: ....

....

Tomorrow's Target
The one thing I want to have achieved by the end of the day tomorrow is: ......

....

Tonight's Thankfulness
Tonight I am thankful for: ....

....

Because: ....

....

Day: ....

Date: ..../........../..........

Morning

Today's word for the day: ....

Today's Target
Today's number one priority I want to achieve is: ....
....

Daily De-stresser
My Daily De-stresser today will be: ....
....

Evening

Big Win
My Big Win today was: ....
....

Because: ....
....

Lesson Learned
Today I learned: ....
....

Happy Highlight
The highlight of my day was: ....
....

Tomorrow's Target
The one thing I want to have achieved by the end of the day tomorrow is: ....
....

Tonight's Thankfulness
Tonight I am thankful for: ....
....

Because: ....
....

My Week In Review

Did I achieve my three WAGs? Circle the appropriate answer

❶ WAG 1:   Yes!   No   (If no, why not): ....

❷ WAG 2   Yes!   No   (If no, why not): ....

❸ WAG 3   Yes!   No   (If no, why not): ....

What was the best unexpected thing that happened to me this week, and why?

What things, if any, didn't go to plan this week?

What actions will I take to avoid this happening again?

What mark out of 10 do I give myself for the past week, and why?

Next week in focus
In a sentence, this is what I want to have achieved by the end of next week, and why:

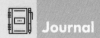

WEEK 8

My Weekly Achievable Goals (WAGs)

My WAGs for this week, to get me one week closer towards achieving my Big Picture Goal, are as follows:

❶ WAG 1:

❷ WAG 2:

❸ WAG 3:

Why are these WAGs so smart?

I have chosen these achievable WAGs for this week for the following reasons:

❶ WAG 1 is a smart weekly goal for me because:

❷ WAG 2 is a smart weekly goal for me because:

❸ WAG 3 is a smart weekly goal for me because:

WEEK 8

This week's Every Day Actions (EDAs)

I will do the following three things every day this week to help me achieve my Weekly Achievable Goals, which will help me achieve my Big Picture Goal:

❶ EDA 1:

❷ EDA 2:

❸ EDA 3:

Tracking my EDAs

	Mon	Tue	Wed	Thur	Fri	Sat	Sun	**Total**	**Goal hit?**
❶ EDA 1									
❷ EDA 2									
❸ EDA 3									

My week in five words

Here I choose five words that describe how achieving this week's WAGs and EDAs will make me feel:

Day: ....

Date: .... / .... / ....

Morning

Today's word for the day: ....

Today's Target
Today's number one priority I want to achieve is: ....
....

Daily De-stresser
My Daily De-stresser today will be: ....
....

Evening

Big Win
My Big Win today was: ....
....

Because: ....
....

Lesson Learned
Today I learned: ....
....

Happy Highlight
The highlight of my day was: ....
....

Tomorrow's Target
The one thing I want to have achieved by the end of the day tomorrow is: ....
....

Tonight's Thankfulness
Tonight I am thankful for: ....
....

Because: ....
....

Day: ....

Date: .... / .... / ....

Morning
Today's word for the day: ....

Today's Target
Today's number one priority I want to achieve is: ....
....

Daily De-stresser
My Daily De-stresser today will be: ....
....

Evening

Big Win
My Big Win today was: ....
....

Because: ....
....

Lesson Learned
Today I learned: ....
....

Happy Highlight
The highlight of my day was: ....
....

Tomorrow's Target
The one thing I want to have achieved by the end of the day tomorrow is: ....
....

Tonight's Thankfulness
Tonight I am thankful for: ....
....

Because: ....
....

Day: _____

Date: _____ / _____ / _____

Morning
Today's word for the day: _____

Today's Target
Today's number one priority I want to achieve is: _____

Daily De-stresser
My Daily De-stresser today will be: _____

Evening

Big Win
My Big Win today was: _____

Because: _____

Lesson Learned
Today I learned: _____

Happy Highlight
The highlight of my day was: _____

Tomorrow's Target
The one thing I want to have achieved by the end of the day tomorrow is: _____

Tonight's Thankfulness
Tonight I am thankful for: _____

Because: _____

Day: ....

Date: .... / .... / ....

Morning
Today's word for the day: ....

Today's Target
Today's number one priority I want to achieve is: ....
....

Daily De-stresser
My Daily De-stresser today will be: ....
....

Evening

Big Win
My Big Win today was: ....
....

Because: ....
....

Lesson Learned
Today I learned: ....
....

Happy Highlight
The highlight of my day was: ....
....

Tomorrow's Target
The one thing I want to have achieved by the end of the day tomorrow is: ....
....

Tonight's Thankfulness
Tonight I am thankful for: ....
....

Because: ....
....

Day: ....

Date: .... / .... / ....

Morning
Today's word for the day: ....

Today's Target
Today's number one priority I want to achieve is: ....
....

Daily De-stresser
My Daily De-stresser today will be: ....
....

Evening

Big Win
My Big Win today was: ....
....

Because: ....
....

Lesson Learned
Today I learned: ....
....

Happy Highlight
The highlight of my day was: ....
....

Tomorrow's Target
The one thing I want to have achieved by the end of the day tomorrow is: ....
....

Tonight's Thankfulness
Tonight I am thankful for: ....
....

Because: ....
....

Day: ....

Date: .... / .... / ....

Morning
Today's word for the day: ....

Today's Target
Today's number one priority I want to achieve is: ....
....

Daily De-stresser
My Daily De-stresser today will be: ....
....

Evening

Big Win
My Big Win today was: ....
....

Because: ....
....

Lesson Learned
Today I learned: ....
....

Happy Highlight
The highlight of my day was: ....
....

Tomorrow's Target
The one thing I want to have achieved by the end of the day tomorrow is: ....
....

Tonight's Thankfulness
Tonight I am thankful for: ....
....

Because: ....
....

Day: ....

Date: .... / .... / ....

Morning
Today's word for the day: ....

Today's Target
Today's number one priority I want to achieve is: ....
....

Daily De-stresser
My Daily De-stresser today will be: ....
....

Evening

Big Win
My Big Win today was: ....
....

Because: ....
....

Lesson Learned
Today I learned: ....
....

Happy Highlight
The highlight of my day was: ....
....

Tomorrow's Target
The one thing I want to have achieved by the end of the day tomorrow is: ....
....

Tonight's Thankfulness
Tonight I am thankful for: ....
....

Because: ....
....

My Week In Review

Did I achieve my three WAGs? Circle the appropriate answer

❶ WAG 1: Yes! No (If no, why not): ....

❷ WAG 2 Yes! No (If no, why not): ....

❸ WAG 3 Yes! No (If no, why not): ....

What was the best unexpected thing that happened to me this week, and why?

....

....

What things, if any, didn't go to plan this week?

....

....

What actions will I take to avoid this happening again?

....

....

What mark out of 10 do I give myself for the past week, and why?

....

....

Next week in focus
In a sentence, this is what I want to have achieved by the end of next week, and why:

....

....

....

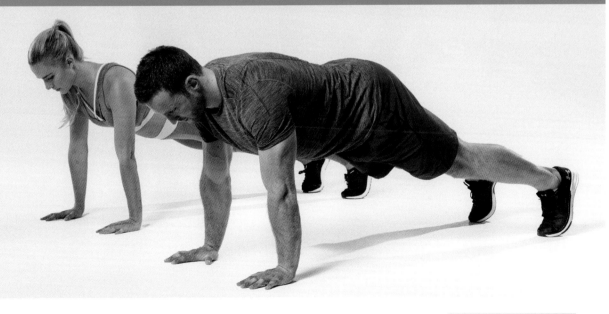

Train smart

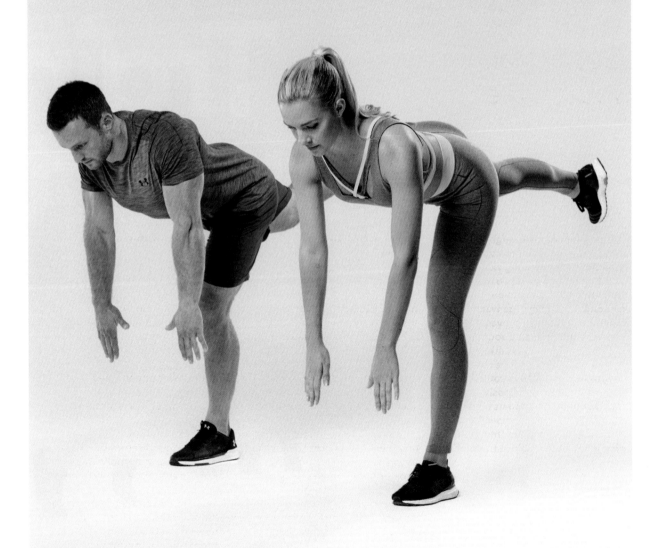

Lose body fat fast!

Get leaner, healthier and happier with your new eight-week exercise plan

It is possible to lose weight by making smart changes to your diet alone – but adding exercise into the mix will help you lose fat much faster, and give you strong and defined muscles as well! More than that, research proves that regular exercise is as good for your mental health as your physical health, helping to reduce anxiety, depression and other problems, and increasing feelings of positivity, motivation and happiness. That's why it's time to start moving your body more – and our eight-week plan is the perfect place to start!

Functional fat loss

This chapter contains your new eight-week fat loss plan, which is based on a principle called high-intensity functional training or HIFT. Research shows HIFT is a superior way of burning fat and defining muscles to high-intensity interval training (HIIT) or low-intensity steady-state cardio, such as jogging.

All the exercises have been selected because they work your muscles through all the main movement patterns in a functional way (hence the name). This will not only help you burn fat, but also get defined muscles and improve your strength, mobility and flexibility, so you move through every day life with ease and without aches and pains.

.

Losing fat made easy

As we explained in the first chapter, one of the best things about your new eight-week exercise plan is that it's so easy to understand and follow – plus you don't need any equipment, so you can do your sessions at home, outside or anywhere with a little bit of space! The sessions don't take long, but each one has been structured to maximise the amount of fat you burn – and accelerate your health and happiness gains – in the minimal amount of time.

There are three workouts per week for the next eight weeks. Each one is made up of different exercises in a circuit, and you'll do a set number of circuits per session. It's really simple, even if you've never done this type of training before, and everything you need to know is clearly explained at the start of each week's programme.

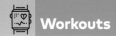

Your week 1 workouts
Your eight-week exercise plan for a leaner and fitter body starts now!

You're now ready to begin your new fat-burning, muscle-defining exercise plan – and getting started couldn't be easier! Here's all you need to know about this week's workouts, followed by a clear breakdown of the three circuit sessions you're going to do this week to turn your body into a fat-burning machine...

This week's workouts

In this first week, as in every week of this plan, you'll do three sessions. Try to leave at least one day between your workouts, so exercising on Monday, Wednesday and Friday is a great way to do it.

All three sessions this week are made up of three circuits of eight different exercises. The guide to doing each exercise can be found by turning to the page number next to the move. The main differences between the sessions this week are how long you do each move and how long you rest before starting the next move in the circuit.

Make sure you warm up before starting each session of the plan. The warm-up is included in the Workout Details table at the top of each page. You'll find further instructions on how to warm up on p226.

Work versus rest

In workouts 1 and 3 you'll follow a 40-20 work-rest split, which means you'll do 40 seconds of exercise 1, rest for 20 seconds, then do exercise 2 for 40 seconds, and so on until you've done 40 seconds of exercise 8. At that point you'll rest for 60 seconds, then repeat the circuit until you've done it a total of three times.

In workout 2 you'll follow a 30-30 work-rest split, which means you'll do 30 seconds of exercise 1, rest for 30 seconds, then do exercise 2 for 30 seconds, and so on until you've done 30 seconds of exercise 8. At that point you'll rest for 60 seconds then repeat the circuit until you've done it three times. And that's it! It really is that easy!

Ready? Let's do this!

WORKOUT DETAILS

Warm-up	**5 minutes**
Total number of circuits	**3**
Work	**40 seconds on**
Rest	**20 seconds off**
Rest between circuits	**60 seconds**

THE CIRCUIT PLAN

Order	Exercise name	Form guide
1	**Chair squat**	p238
2	**Chair dip bent knees**	p237
3	**Lunge**	p245
4	**Glute bridge**	p240
5	**Standing sprint**	p258
6	**Pogo**	p249
7	**Bicycle**	p235
8	**Plank**	p248
Rest	**60 seconds**	

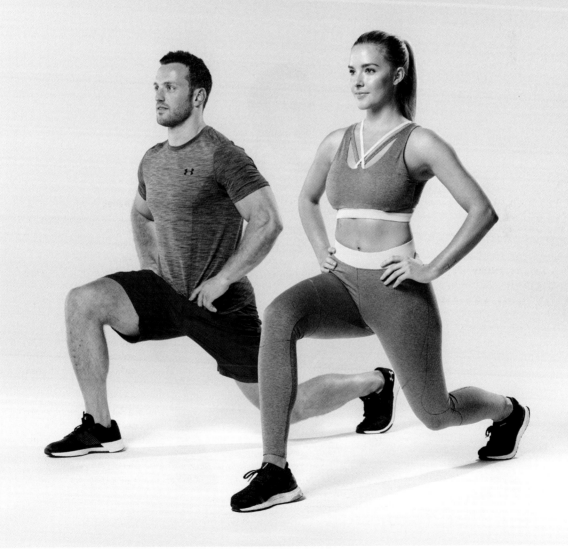

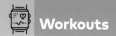
Week 1 • Workout 2

WORKOUT DETAILS

Warm-up	**5 minutes**
Total number of circuits	**3**
Work	**30 seconds on**
Rest	**30 seconds off**
Rest between circuits	**60 seconds**

THE CIRCUIT PLAN

Order	Exercise name	Form guide
1	**Squat**	p256
2	**Press-up knees-up**	p250
3	**Reverse lunge**	p251
4	**Diagonal mountain climber**	p239
5	**High knees**	p241
6	**Butt kick**	p236
7	**Standing Russian twist**	p258
8	**Leg raise hold**	p245
Rest	**60 seconds**	

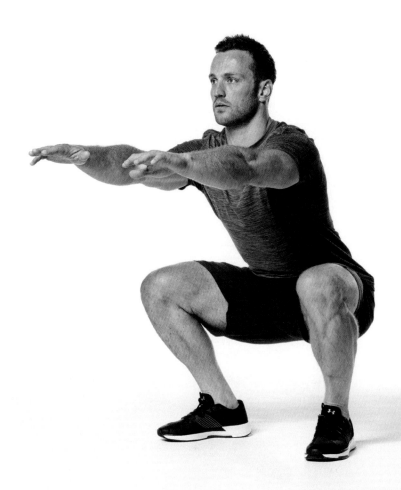

WORKOUT DETAILS

Warm-up	**5 minutes**
Total number of circuits	**3**
Work	**40 seconds on**
Rest	**20 seconds off**
Rest between circuits	**60 seconds**

THE CIRCUIT PLAN

Order	Exercise name	Form guide
1	**Overhead squat**	p247
2	**Chair press-up**	p237
3	**Curtsy lunge**	p238
4	**Romanian deadlift**	p252
5	**Walking down-up**	p265
6	**Star jump**	p259
7	**Rolling plank**	p251
8	**Arch hold**	p234
Rest	**60 seconds**	

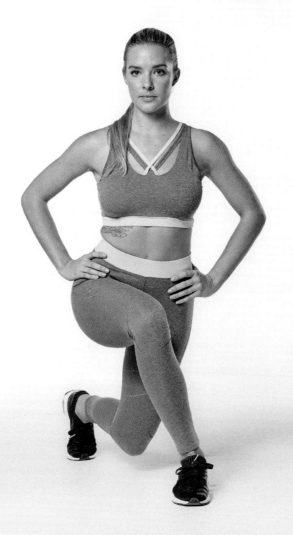

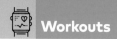
Your week 2 workouts

Keep up your new exercise habit this week and watch the weight fall off!

Now that your three week 1 workouts are in the bag, you should already be feeling a little fitter and healthier, and raring to get week 2 started to keep the positive results coming! There's a few simple but important changes to your workouts this week to keep them challenging to help your body burn fat faster. But don't worry – you've already done week 1 and in many ways that's the hardest, especially if you are new to this type of training. Now you're up and running, stay positive and confident and you'll take another big step forwards this week towards a leaner, healthier and happier life!

This week's workouts
Just like last week, there are three sessions this week. Try to leave at least one day between your workouts, so again, Monday, Wednesday and Friday is a great approach. Again, all three workouts are made up of eight different exercises, but this week the number of total circuits and the time you work and rest change so you challenge your body a little bit more. Why? That's the quickest and best way to get leaner and healthier!

Work versus rest
In workouts 1 and 3 you'll follow a 20-10 work-rest split, which means you'll do 20 seconds of exercise 1, rest for 10 seconds, then do exercise 2 for 20 seconds, and so on until you've done 20 seconds of exercise 8. At that point you'll rest for 60 seconds, then repeat the circuit until you've done it a total of six times.

In workout 2 you'll follow a 30-30 work-rest split, which means you'll do 30 seconds of exercise 1, rest for 30 seconds, then do exercise 2 for 30 seconds, and so on until you've done 30 seconds of exercise 8. At that point you'll rest for 60 seconds, then repeat the circuit until you've done it three times. Make sure you do the full warm-up routine before starting each session.

WORKOUT DETAILS

Warm-up	**5 minutes**
Total number of circuits	**6**
Work	**20 seconds on**
Rest	**10 seconds off**
Rest between circuits	**60 seconds**

THE CIRCUIT PLAN

Order	Exercise name	Form guide
1	**Sumo squat**	p259
2	**Press-up**	p249
3	**Rotating lunge**	p252
4	**Romanian deadlift**	p252
5	**Squat jump**	p257
6	**Plank jack**	p248
7	**Tall plank shoulder tap**	p261
8	**Leg raise**	p244
Rest	**60 seconds**	

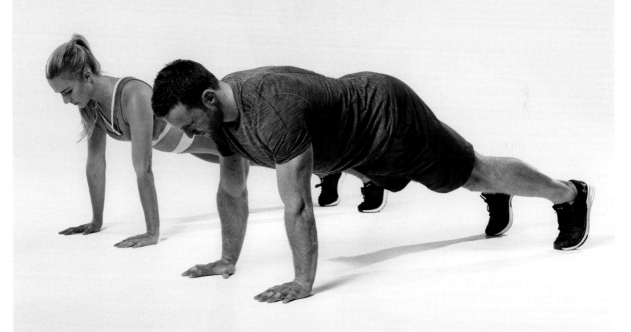

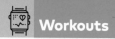

Week 2 • Workout 2

WORKOUT DETAILS

Warm-up	**5 minutes**
Total number of circuits	**3**
Work	**30 seconds on**
Rest	**30 seconds off**
Rest between circuits	**60 seconds**

THE CIRCUIT PLAN

Order	Exercise name	Form guide
1	**Prisoner squat**	p251
2	**Chair dip straight legs**	p237
3	**Prisoner lunge**	p250
4	**Marching glute bridge**	p246
5	**Standing sprint**	p258
6	**Speed skater**	p255
7	**Heel touch**	p241
8	**Tall plank**	p260
Rest	**60 seconds**	

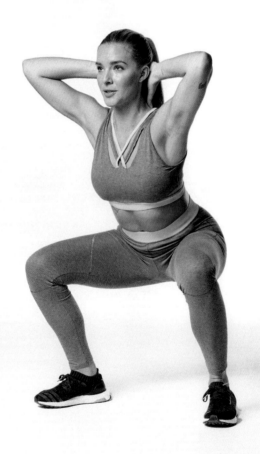

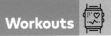
Week 2 • Workout 3

WORKOUT DETAILS

Warm-up	**5 minutes**
Total number of circuits	**6**
Work	**20 seconds on**
Rest	**10 seconds off**
Rest between circuits	**60 seconds**

THE CIRCUIT PLAN

Order	Exercise name	Form guide
1	**Two-pulse squat**	p264
2	**Chair press-up**	p237
3	**Side lunge**	p253
4	**Crunch**	p238
5	**Down-up**	p239
6	**Mountain climber**	p246
7	**Tall plank toe tap**	p261
8	**Hollow body**	p242
Rest	**60 seconds**	

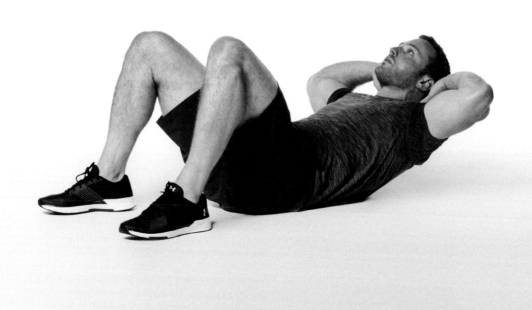

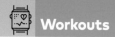

Your week 3 workouts

Stay focused on your better-body mission to keep getting fitter!

You're now about to start week 3 of your fat-torching exercise plan, which means you're already 25% of the way through the eight-week plan. Time flies when you're losing fat! But we want your results to get even better, so with that in mind there are some changes to the three workouts this week – designed to keep your body in that fat-burning mode you want!

This week's workouts
Like every week in this eight-week plan there are three sessions this week and, as always, you should try to leave at least one day between workouts, rather than do all three sessions on consecutive days. That approach means you'll go four full days without exercising, which is far from ideal in terms of maximising fat loss and improving health and fitness, and also won't help to make exercise one of your new healthy habits!

The biggest change this week is that the number of moves in each circuit increases by one, so there are now nine exercises. The work-versus-rest periods remain in a familiar ratio to help you burn body fat fast!

Work versus rest
In workouts 1 and 3 you'll follow a 45-15 work-rest split, which means you'll do 45 seconds of exercise 1, rest for 15 seconds, then do exercise 2 for 45 seconds, and so on until you've done 45 seconds of exercise 9. At that point you'll rest for 60 seconds, then repeat the circuit until you've done it a total of three times.

In workout 2 you'll follow a 40-20 work-rest split, which means you'll do 40 seconds of exercise 1, rest for 20 seconds, then do exercise 2 for 40 seconds, and so on until you've done 40 seconds of exercise 9. At that point you'll rest for 60 seconds, then repeat the circuit until you've done it four times.

Remember to warm up before each session (see p226) to prepare your mind and your muscles for the workout ahead!

Week 3 • Workout 1

WORKOUT DETAILS

Warm-up	**5 minutes**
Total number of circuits	**3**
Work	**45 seconds on**
Rest	**15 seconds off**
Rest between circuits	**60 seconds**

THE CIRCUIT PLAN

Order	Exercise name	Form guide
1	**Star jump**	p259
2	**Squat**	p256
3	**Lunge with arm raise**	p245
4	**Two-to-one jump**	p265
5	**Hands-up press-up**	p241
6	**Mountain climber**	p246
7	**Static bear crawl**	p259
8	**Half Turkish get-up**	p240
9	**Squat hold**	p257
Rest	**60 seconds**	

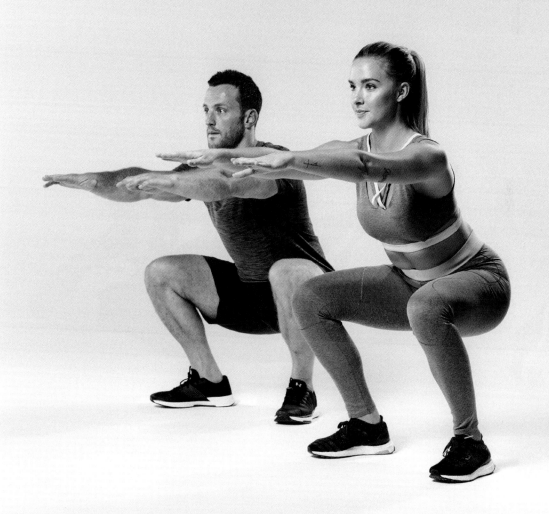

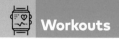

Week 3 • Workout 2

WORKOUT DETAILS

Warm-up	**5 minutes**
Total number of circuits	**4**
Work	**40 seconds on**
Rest	**20 seconds off**
Rest between circuits	**60 seconds**

THE CIRCUIT PLAN

Order	Exercise name	Form guide
1	**Sumo squat**	p259
2	**Side lunge**	p253
3	**Glute bridge**	p240
4	**Press-up knees-up**	p250
5	**Three-pulse squat**	p263
6	**Overhead reverse lunge**	p247
7	**Jackknife**	p242
8	**Bicycle**	p235
9	**Plank**	p248
Rest	**60 seconds**	

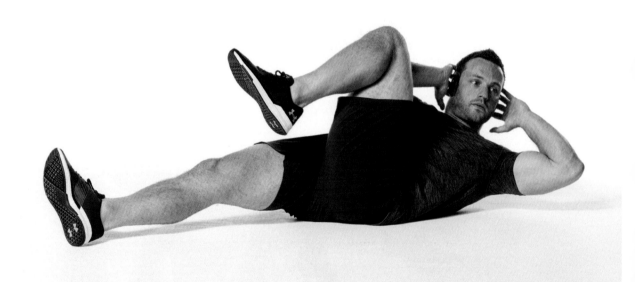

Week 3 • Workout 3

WORKOUT DETAILS

Warm-up	**5 minutes**
Total number of circuits	**3**
Work	**45 seconds on**
Rest	**15 seconds off**
Rest between circuits	**60 seconds**

THE CIRCUIT PLAN

Order	Exercise name	Form guide
1	**Standing sprint**	p258
2	**Overhead squat**	p247
3	**Lean-over lunge**	p244
4	**Tuck jump**	p264
5	**Pike**	p248
6	**Chair dip straight legs**	p237
7	**Burpee**	p236
8	**Thread the needle**	p263
9	**Leg raise**	p244
Rest	**60 seconds**	

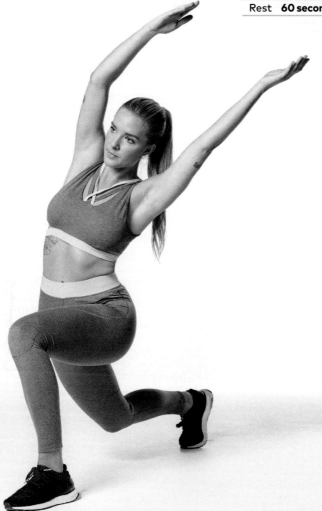

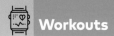

Your week 4 workouts

More work and less rest is the key this week to unlock faster fat loss!

At the end of this week you will be halfway through this plan and by now you should be feeling leaner, healthier and fitter! The good news is this week will keep the great results coming because while the following three sessions are very similar to the previous week, they are a little bit harder thanks to longer work periods and shorter rest periods that'll force your body to release more stored fat for fuel. Remember, every rep counts in the fight against fat!

This week's workouts
Like last week there are three sessions this week, and all three are made up of circuits of nine different exercises.

Now that you are becoming very familiar with the exercises in this plan, and how the circuits work, try to focus on moving as quickly as possible between the different moves in each circuit. The less time you spend resting the more time you spend working, and getting your heart rate high and getting hot and sweaty are the perfect signs that your effort is going to make your body leaner and fitter!

Work versus rest
In workouts 1 and 3 you'll follow a 50-10 work-rest split, which means you'll do 50 seconds of exercise 1, rest for 10 seconds, then do exercise 2 for 50 seconds, and so on until you've done 50 seconds of exercise 9. At that point you'll rest for 60 seconds, then repeat the circuit until you've done it a total of three times.

In workout 2 you'll follow a 40-20 work-rest split, which means you'll do 40 seconds of exercise 1, rest for 20 seconds, then do exercise 2 for 40 seconds, and so on until you've done 40 seconds of exercise 9. At that point you'll rest for 60 seconds, then repeat the circuit until you've done it four times.

As always, it's really important to warm up (p226) before each session – and doing so will help you burn even more body fat!

WORKOUT DETAILS

Warm-up	**5 minutes**
Total number of circuits	**3**
Work	**50 seconds on**
Rest	**10 seconds off**
Rest between circuits	**60 seconds**

THE CIRCUIT PLAN

Order	Exercise name	Form guide
1	**Pogo**	p249
2	**Two-pulse squat**	p264
3	**Rotating lunge**	p252
4	**Standing sprint**	p258
5	**Alternating toe touch**	p234
6	**Offset press-up**	p246
7	**Burpee**	p236
8	**Seated Russian twist**	p253
9	**Plank**	p248
Rest	**60 seconds**	

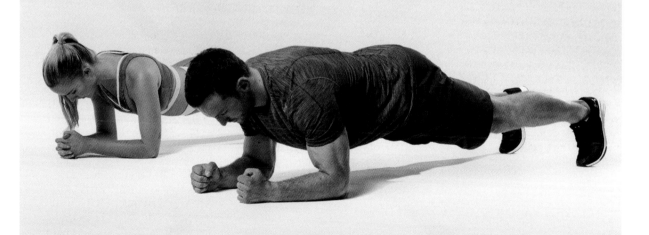

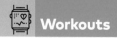
Week 4 • Workout 2

WORKOUT DETAILS

Warm-up	**5 minutes**
Total number of circuits	**4**
Work	**40 seconds on**
Rest	**20 seconds off**
Rest between circuits	**60 seconds**

THE CIRCUIT PLAN

Order	Exercise name	Form guide
1	**Overhead squat**	p247
2	**Transverse lunge**	p263
3	**Romanian deadlift**	p252
4	**Press-up**	p249
5	**Split squat**	p256
6	**Side lunge**	p253
7	**Single-leg glute bridge**	p254
8	**Rolling plank**	p251
9	**Side plank**	p253
Rest	**60 seconds**	

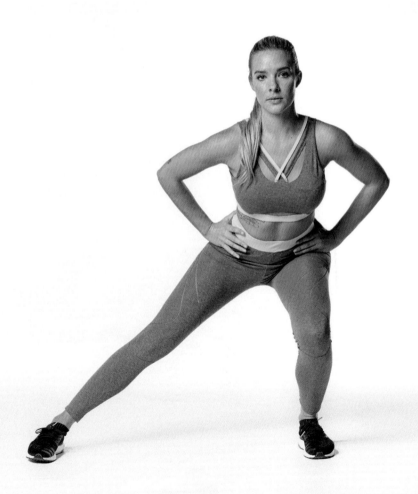

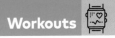
WORKOUT DETAILS

Warm-up	**5 minutes**
Total number of circuits	**3**
Work	**50 seconds on**
Rest	**10 seconds off**
Rest between circuits	**60 seconds**

THE CIRCUIT PLAN

Order	Exercise name	Form guide
1	**Lateral jump**	p243
2	**Three-pulse squat**	p263
3	**Lean-over lunge**	p244
4	**Speed skater**	p255
5	**Jackknife**	p242
6	**Chair dip bent knees**	p237
7	**Squat thrust**	p257
8	**Thread the needle**	p263
9	**Hollow body**	p242
Rest	**60 seconds**	

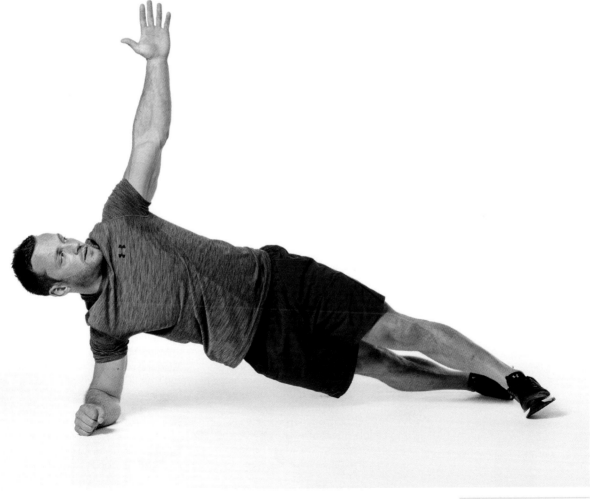

Your week 5 workouts

You're halfway through the plan: let's kick on to keep the results coming!

You're already halfway through the eight-week plan and should have noticed some big changes to how you look in the mirror and how your clothes fit – and, just as importantly, some big changes to the way you feel! And now it's time to push on into the final half of the plan to ensure you get the best possible fat loss results.

This week's workouts

There are three sessions this week again and, as usual, you should try to leave a day between workouts for the best results. However, there is one significant change this week – the circuits have been changed to make them slightly more challenging to help you get the results you want faster.

All three sessions this week are made up of nine exercises, split into three mini-circuits that come together to form one complete circuit. This means you'll do the first three moves in a mini-circuit three times before moving on to the next three moves, and then the same for the final three moves in the workout.

This approach makes this week tough, but that's what it takes to make big and positive changes to the way you look and feel!

Work versus rest

In workouts 1 and 3 you'll follow a 60-0 work-rest split, which means you'll do 60 seconds of exercise 1A, then go straight into 60 seconds of 1B, then straight into 60 seconds of 1C. Only then do you rest, for 60 seconds, before going back to 1A and repeating this pattern until you've done it a total of three times. You then follow the same pattern with 2A, 2B and 2C, doing this mini-circuit three times, before finishing the workout with three mini-circuits of 3A, 3B and 3C.

In workout 2 you'll follow a 30-30 work-rest split, which means you'll do 30 seconds of exercise 1A, rest for 30 seconds, then do move 1B for 30 seconds, rest for 30 seconds, and then 1C for 30 seconds, then rest for 60 seconds. You'll do this mini-circuit three times, then repeat this pattern with moves 2A, 2B and 2C, and then finish the workout with three mini-circuits of moves 3A, 3B and 3C.

WORKOUT DETAILS

Warm-up	**5 minutes**
Total number of circuits	**3**
Work	**60 seconds on**
Rest	**0 seconds off**
Rest between mini-circuits	**60 seconds**

THE CIRCUIT PLAN

Order	Exercise name	Form guide
1A	**Squat**	p256
1B	**Reverse lunge**	p251
1C	**Marching glute bridge**	p246
Rest	**60 seconds**	
2A	**Chair press-up**	p237
2B	**Single-leg Romanian deadlift**	p254
2C	**Two-to-one jump**	p265
Rest	**60 seconds**	
3A	**Single-leg Russian twist**	p255
3B	**Plank**	p248
3C	**Bear crawl**	p234
Rest	**60 seconds**	

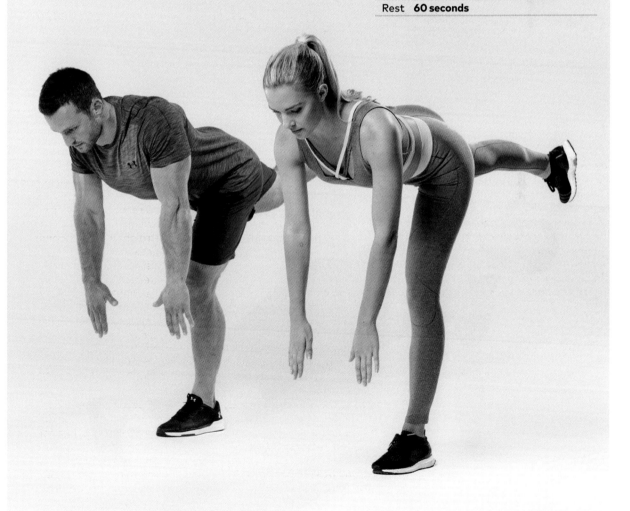

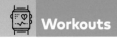

Week 5 • Workout 2

WORKOUT DETAILS

Warm-up	**5 minutes**
Total number of circuits	**3**
Work	**30 seconds on**
Rest	**30 seconds off**
Rest between mini-circuits	**60 seconds**

THE CIRCUIT PLAN

Order	Exercise name	Form guide
1A	**Sumo squat**	p259
1B	**Curtsy lunge**	p238
1C	**Pogo**	p249
Rest	**60 seconds**	
2A	**Squat jump**	p257
2B	**T press-up**	p260
2C	**Lateral jump**	p243
Rest	**60 seconds**	
3A	**Crunch**	p238
3B	**Tall plank shoulder tap**	p261
3C	**Hollow body**	p242
Rest	**60 seconds**	

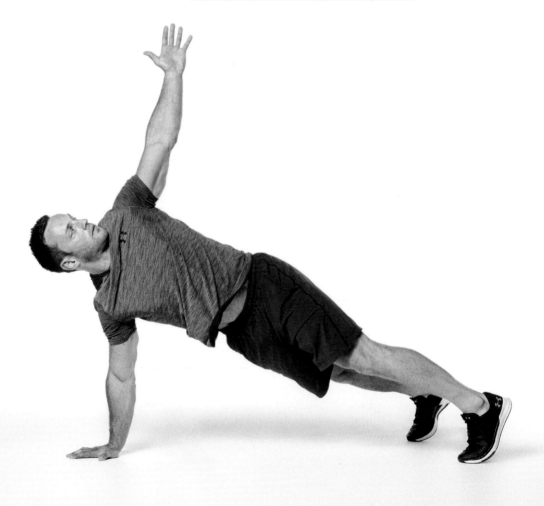

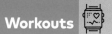
Week 5 • Workout 3

WORKOUT DETAILS

Warm-up	**5 minutes**
Total number of circuits	**3**
Work	**60 seconds on**
Rest	**0 seconds off**
Rest between mini-circuits	**60 seconds**

THE CIRCUIT PLAN

Order	Exercise name	Form guide
1A	**Split squat**	p256
1B	**Prisoner lunge**	p250
1C	**Mountain climber**	p246
Rest	**60 seconds**	
2A	**Press-up knees-up**	p250
2B	**Romanian deadlift**	p252
2C	**Lateral bear crawl**	p242
Rest	**60 seconds**	
3A	**Heel touch**	p241
3B	**Diagonal mountain climber**	p239
3C	**Plank jack**	p248
Rest	**60 seconds**	

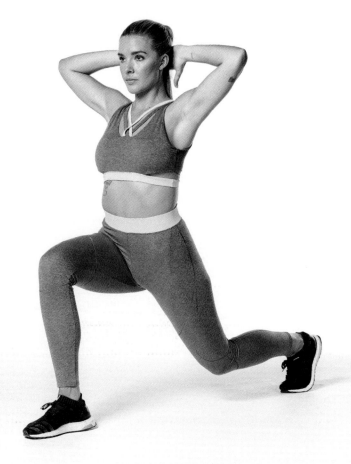

Your week 6 workouts

Every bit of extra effort this week will help you get the best possible results!

There's only three weeks of the plan – or just nine sessions – left, so now's the time to really push yourself harder than ever before! If until now you've been a bit relaxed about sticking to the precise work-versus-rest splits, try to stick to them exactly as they are detailed to maximise the time you spend working and minimise the time you spend resting. Because the more intensively you work out during these final nine sessions, the more fat you'll burn and the greater your health and fitness results!

This week's workouts
This week's three workouts follow the same new pattern you used in week 5, with the main circuit broken down into three mini-circuits of three moves each. This approach will keep your muscles, and your heart and lungs, working hard to burn body fat quickly!

As always, do a thorough warm-up (see p226) to get your muscles firing for the best possible results.

Work versus rest
In workouts 1 and 3 you'll follow a 40-20 work-rest split, which means you'll do 40 seconds of exercise 1A, rest for 20 seconds, do 40 seconds of 1B, rest for 20 seconds, then 40 seconds of 1C, then rest for 60 seconds. You then go back to 1A and repeat this pattern until you've done it a total of four times. Then follow the same pattern with moves 2A, 2B and 2C, doing this mini-circuit four times, before finishing the workout with four mini-circuits of moves 3A, 3B and 3C.

In workout 2 you'll follow a 60-0 work-rest split, which means you'll do 60 seconds of exercises 1A, 1B and 1C, and then rest for 60 seconds. You'll do this mini-circuit four times, then repeat this pattern four times with moves 2A, 2B and 2C, and then finish the workout with four mini-circuits of moves 3A, 3B and 3C.

Week 6 • Workout 1

WORKOUT DETAILS

Warm-up	**5 minutes**
Total number of circuits	**4**
Work	**40 seconds on**
Rest	**20 seconds off**
Rest between mini-circuits	**60 seconds**

THE CIRCUIT PLAN

Order	Exercise name	Form guide
1A	**Pause squat**	p247
1B	**Rotating reverse lunge**	p252
1C	**Down-up**	p239
Rest	**60 seconds**	
2A	**Press-up**	p249
2B	**Alternating toe touch**	p234
2C	**High knees**	p241
Rest	**60 seconds**	
3A	**Seated Russian twist**	p253
3B	**Plank**	p248
3C	**Burpee**	p236
Rest	**60 seconds**	

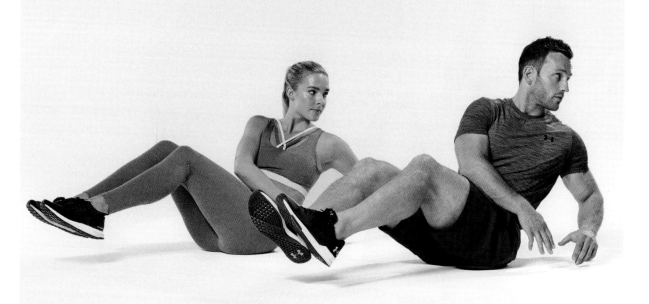

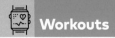
Week 6 • Workout 2

WORKOUT DETAILS

Warm-up	**5 minutes**
Total number of circuits	**4**
Work	**60 seconds on**
Rest	**0 seconds off**
Rest between mini-circuits	**60 seconds**

THE CIRCUIT PLAN

Order	Exercise name	Form guide
1A	**Bulgarian split squat**	p235
1B	**Sumo squat**	p259
1C	**Single-leg glute bridge**	p254
Rest	**60 seconds**	
2A	**Side lunge**	p253
2B	**Tall plank**	p260
2C	**Butt kick**	p236
Rest	**60 seconds**	
3A	**Single-leg Romanian deadlift reach**	p255
3B	**Half Turkish get-up**	p240
3C	**Side plank**	p253
Rest	**60 seconds**	

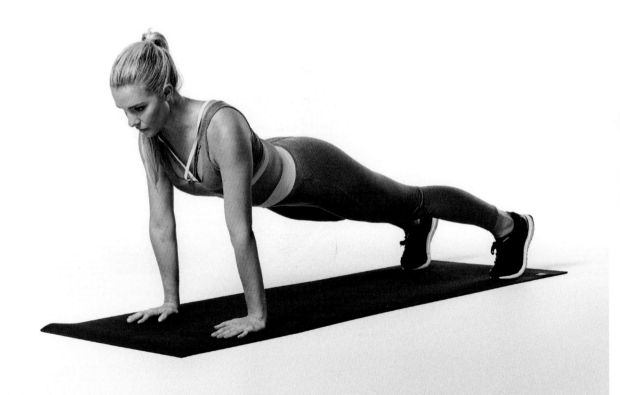

Week 6 • Workout 3

WORKOUT DETAILS

Warm-up	**5 minutes**
Total number of circuits	**4**
Work	**40 seconds on**
Rest	**20 seconds off**
Rest between mini-circuits	**60 seconds**

THE CIRCUIT PLAN

Order	Exercise name	Form guide
1A	**Lunge with arm raise**	p245
1B	**Standing jog**	p258
1C	**Overhead squat**	p247
Rest	**60 seconds**	
2A	**Hands-up press-up**	p241
2B	**Romanian deadlift**	p252
2C	**Standing sprint**	p258
Rest	**60 seconds**	
3A	**Bicycle**	p235
3B	**Arch hold**	p234
3C	**Burpee**	p236
Rest	**60 seconds**	

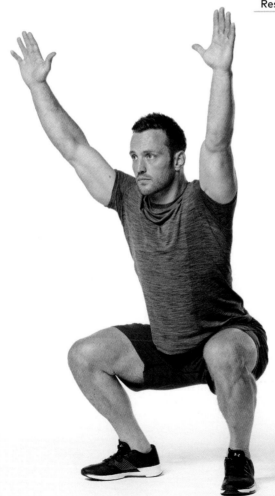

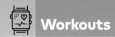
Your week 7 workouts

It's the final fortnight of the plan so dig deep to keep getting leaner!

It's the final two weeks of the plan, and any extra effort you can find now to put into your sessions this week and next week will go a huge way towards turning your good results into great results! Give every workout everything you've got and push harder than ever to give your body the stimulus it needs to keep shifting that fat.

This week's workouts
There are three workouts again this week, and each circuit is made up of two mini-circuits of four moves each. This approach keeps the session short and intense, which is exactly what you need to do to make the biggest and most positive changes to the way you look and feel!

Stick to the exercises in order, and remember to keep your rest periods no longer than is detailed in the tables. The aim is to keep you working hard to lose body fat as effectively and efficiently as possible!

Work versus rest
In workouts 1 and 3 you'll follow a 45-15 work-rest split, which means you'll do 45 seconds of exercise 1A, rest for 15 seconds, do 45 seconds of 1B, rest for 15 seconds, do 45 seconds of 1C, rest for 15 seconds, then do 45 seconds of 1D, then rest for 60 seconds. You then go back to 1A and repeat this pattern until you've done it a total of four times. You then follow the same pattern with moves 2A, 2B, 2C and 2D, doing this mini-circuit four times to complete the workout.

In workout 2 you'll follow a 50-10 work-rest split, which means you'll do 50 seconds of exercise 1A, rest for 10 seconds, then do the same for 1B and 1C, then finally do 50 seconds of 1D, then rest for 60 seconds. You then go back to 1A and repeat this until you've done it four times. You then follow the same pattern with moves 2A, 2B, 2C and 2D, doing this mini-circuit four times to complete the workout.

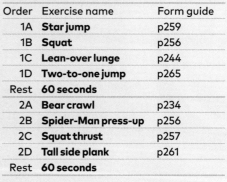

Week 7 • Workout 1

WORKOUT DETAILS

Warm-up	**5 minutes**
Total number of circuits	**4**
Work	**45 seconds on**
Rest	**15 seconds off**
Rest between mini-circuits	**60 seconds**

THE CIRCUIT PLAN

Order	Exercise name	Form guide
1A	**Star jump**	p259
1B	**Squat**	p256
1C	**Lean-over lunge**	p244
1D	**Two-to-one jump**	p265
Rest	**60 seconds**	
2A	**Bear crawl**	p234
2B	**Spider-Man press-up**	p256
2C	**Squat thrust**	p257
2D	**Tall side plank**	p261
Rest	**60 seconds**	

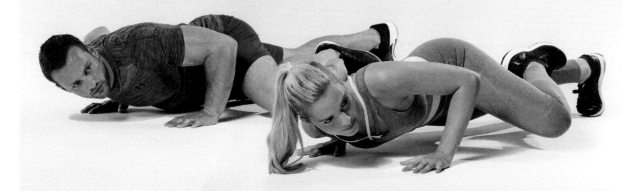

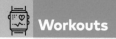
Week 7 • Workout 2

WORKOUT DETAILS

Warm-up	**5 minutes**
Total number of circuits	**4**
Work	**50 seconds on**
Rest	**10 seconds off**
Rest between mini-circuits	**60 seconds**

THE CIRCUIT PLAN

Order	Exercise name	Form guide
1A	**Standing jog**	p258
1B	**Speed skater**	p255
1C	**Butt kick**	p236
1D	**Tuck jump**	p264
Rest	**60 seconds**	
2A	**Single-leg Romanian deadlift**	p254
2B	**Rotating lunge**	p252
2C	**Glute bridge**	p240
2D	**Squat hold**	p257
Rest	**60 seconds**	

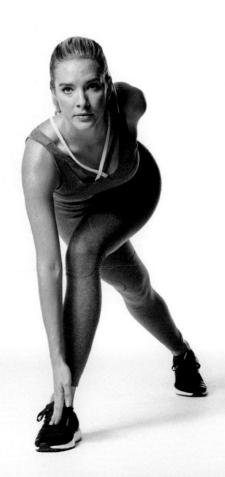

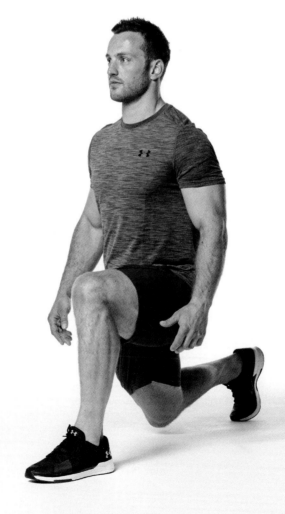

Week 7 • Workout 3

WORKOUT DETAILS

Warm-up	**5 minutes**
Total number of circuits	**4**
Work	**45 seconds on**
Rest	**15 seconds off**
Rest between mini-circuits	**60 seconds**

THE CIRCUIT PLAN

Order	Exercise name	Form guide
1A	**Press-up**	p249
1B	**Squat**	p256
1C	**Romanian deadlift**	p252
1D	**Hollow body**	p242
Rest	**60 seconds**	
2A	**Squat thrust**	p257
2B	**Down-up**	p239
2C	**Lunge**	p245
2D	**Arch hold**	p234
Rest	**60 seconds**	

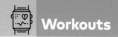
Your week 8 workouts

Give these three sessions all you've got to finish the plan strong!

There may only be three sessions of the plan left, but what you do in this final week will make a huge difference to your final results! You've done so well to get this far, so give it everything you've got each time you train this week to finish the plan leaner, fitter and stronger than you would have ever thought possible.

This week's workouts
In this final week, workouts 1 and 3 are made up of two mini-circuits of three moves each, while workout 2 is made up of two mini-circuits of four moves each.

Just stay focused on performing each of the moves with perfect form, and keep working hard – even when it feels like you want to stop. Every extra rep you can do this week really does add up, and it will all come together to help you finish this eight-week plan in the shape of your life!

Work versus rest
In workouts 1 and 3 you'll follow a 60-0 work-rest split, which means you'll do 60 seconds of exercise 1A, then go straight into 60 seconds of 1B, then straight into 60 seconds of 1C. Only then do you rest, for 60 seconds, before going back to 1A and repeating this pattern until you've done it a total of four times. You then follow exactly the same pattern with moves 2A, 2B and 2C, doing this mini-circuit four times to complete the workout.

In workout 2 you'll follow a 30-30 work-rest split, which means you'll do 30 seconds of exercise 1A, rest for 30 seconds, then do the same for 1B and 1C, then finally do 30 seconds of 1D, then rest for 60 seconds. You'll then do this mini-circuit four times, then repeat this pattern with exercises 2A, 2B, 2C and 2D until you've done it four times to complete the workout.

WORKOUT DETAILS

Warm-up	**5 minutes**
Total number of circuits	**4**
Work	**60 seconds on**
Rest	**0 seconds off**
Rest between mini-circuits	**60 seconds**

THE CIRCUIT PLAN

Order	Exercise name	Form guide
1A	**Turkish get-up**	p262
1B	**Tall plank**	p260
1C	**Single-leg hollow body**	p254
Rest	**60 seconds**	
2A	**Lateral press-up**	p243
2B	**Lean-over reverse lunge**	p244
2C	**Burpee**	p236
Rest	**60 seconds**	

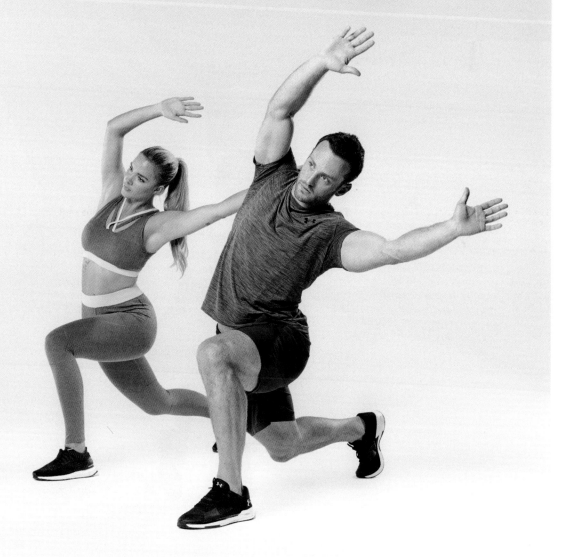

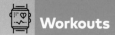
Week 8 • Workout 2

WORKOUT DETAILS

Warm-up	**5 minutes**
Total number of circuits	**4**
Work	**30 seconds on**
Rest	**30 seconds off**
Rest between mini-circuits	**60 seconds**

THE CIRCUIT PLAN

Order	Exercise name	Form guide
1A	**Three-pulse squat**	p263
1B	**Lateral jump**	p243
1C	**Squat jump**	p257
1D	**Squat thrust**	p257
Rest	**60 seconds**	
2A	**Jackknife**	p242
2B	**Plank jack**	p248
2C	**Thread the needle**	p263
2D	**Tuck jump**	p264
Rest	**60 seconds**	

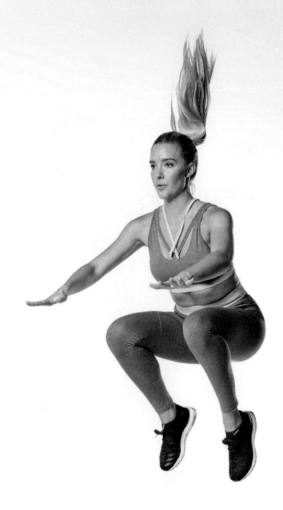

WORKOUT DETAILS

Warm-up	**5 minutes**
Total number of circuits	**4**
Work	**60 seconds on**
Rest	**0 seconds off**
Rest between mini-circuits	**60 seconds**

THE CIRCUIT PLAN

Order	Exercise name	Form guide
1A	**Hands-up press-up**	p241
1B	**Overhead squat**	p247
1C	**Speed skater**	p255
Rest	**60 seconds**	
2A	**Side lunge**	p253
2B	**Tall plank shoulder tap**	p261
2C	**Crunch**	p238
Rest	**60 seconds**	

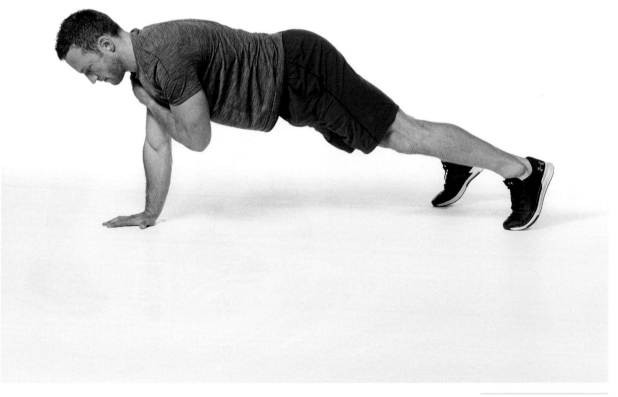

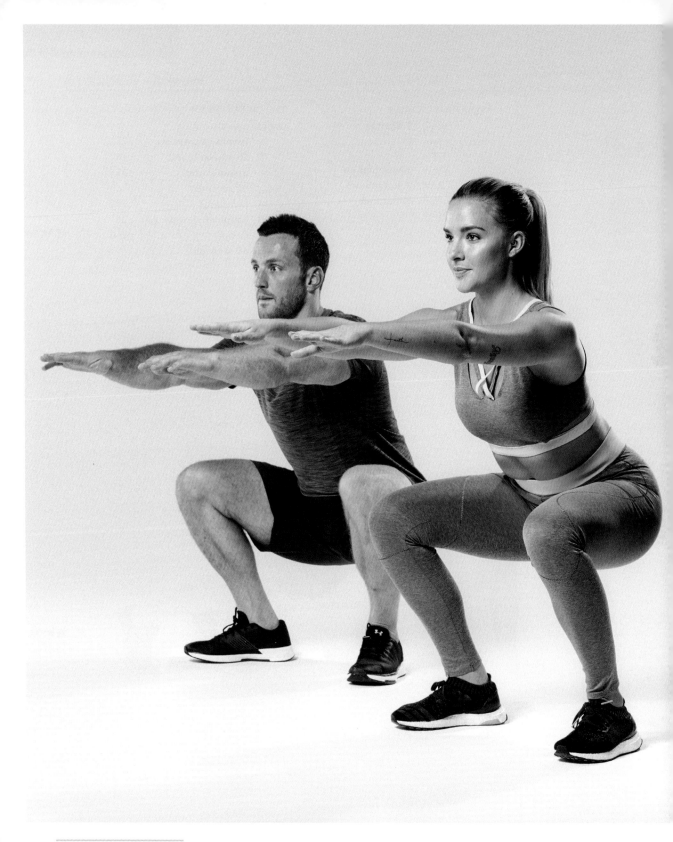

Form guide

How to do the moves

Here's how to warm up, perform the exercises perfectly, and stretch for a better body

To lose body fat and build defined muscles for a leaner, stronger and healthier body, you need to follow the workout plan that begins on p187. And by following the advice ahead, you'll learn how to warm up properly, how to do each exercise with fantastic form for faster results, and how to stretch your muscles effectively to keep your body injury-free and moving well!

Warm-up and stretching
Starting on p226 you'll find the quick and easy warm-up routine to do before each session. It's really important that you do this quick warm-up because it helps your mind and muscles go from a resting state to an active state so you can push yourself hard without the risk of injury.

A warm-up prepares your body by gradually increasing your heart rate, raising your body temperature and making your muscles more flexible and your joints more mobile. It also focuses your mind on the session ahead, blocking out any stresses or worries so you can visualise how good this session is going to go, and how much better you're going to feel once you've done it!

After your session it's just as important to give your body some time to go back to its resting state after being active. You can do this by taking some deep breaths and doing some static-hold stretching to lower your heart rate and improve the flexibility and mobility of your muscles and joints, which is essential to moving better and staying free from injury and pain.

After exercise is the best time for static stretching because your muscles are warm and pliable, allowing you to get into and hold deeper stretches. Find our guide to smarter stretching on p230, and remember not to hold your breath! Breathing deeply and slowly will lower your heart rate and help you hold those deeper stretches.

The exercises
From p234 we list all the moves in the plan alphabetically so you know how to perform them perfectly, which will make them even more effective. Each move is demonstrated with photos and form guides. Follow the instructions and start shifting fat fast!

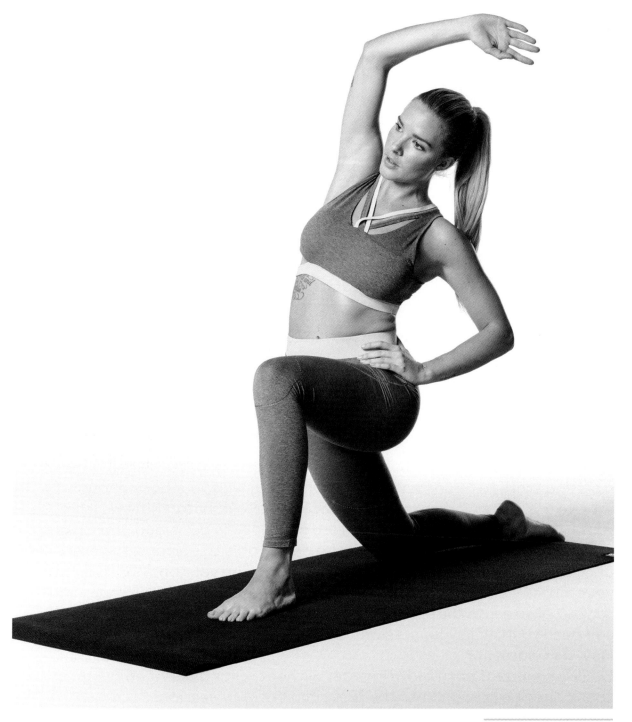

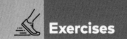

Warm up your body

Do this quick warm-up before every session to prepare your muscles and your mind!

A warm-up prepares your body for physical activity, because going from a resting state to a very active state without giving your body enough time to adjust can increase your risk of injury. So it's vital that you increase your heart rate and body temperature gradually to get blood and oxygen flowing to your muscles, making them better able to perform the exercises ahead without any problems. As well as preparing your body by making your muscles and joints more mobile, a warm-up also focuses your mind so you can execute the exercises as well as possible – and the harder you can push yourself in your sessions, the better your fat loss results will be!

How do I warm up?

Do 30 seconds of each move in order without resting between them. Then go straight into the first circuit of your session.

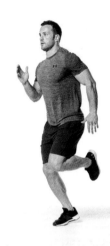

Standing jog

- Stand tall with your chest up and abs engaged.

- Jog on the spot, swinging your arms back and forth.

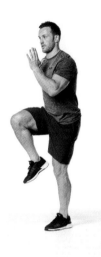

Squat

- Stand tall with your chest up, abs engaged and arms straight by your sides.

- Bend your knees to squat down as low as you can.

- Push through your heels to straighten your legs and return to the start position.

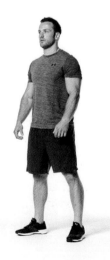

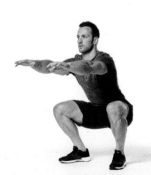

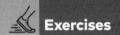
Lunge rotation

- Stand tall with your chest up, abs engaged and arms straight out in front of you.

- Take a big step forwards with your left foot, then bend both knees to lunge down while rotating your torso to your left.

- Push through your front foot to return to the start, then step forwards with your right foot and repeat the move, rotating your torso to the right.

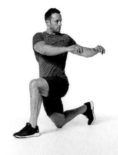
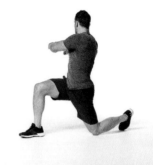

Downward dog

- Start on all fours with straight arms and legs and your hips raised as high as possible.

- Lower your hips to the floor while raising your torso off the floor.

- Raise your hips again to return to the start.

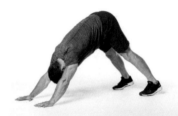
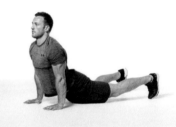

Cat to camel

- Start on your hands and knees with your head raised, looking upwards.

- Lower your head while raising your upper back.

- Lower your upper back to return to the start.

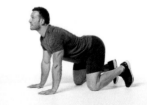
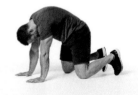

T-rotation

- Start on your hands and knees then straighten one leg and reach out to the side with it.

- Bend the arm on that side so your fingers touch the side of your head.

- Rotate inwards so your elbow touches your other arm then rotate your torso to raise that elbow as high as possible.

- Return to the start and repeat on the other side.

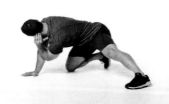 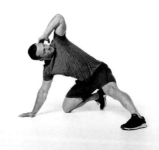

High knees

- Stand tall with your chest up and abs engaged.

- Start sprinting on the spot, swinging your arms and bringing your knees up as high as possible.

- You can also put your arms out straight in front of you and try to make your knees hit your palms with each step.

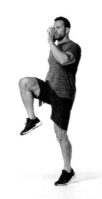 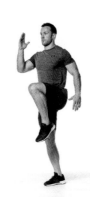

Star jump

- Stand tall with your chest up, abs engaged and hands by your sides.

- Jump up and bring both feet out wide to the sides while raising your arms to the sides so your hands finish above your head.

- Jump back from the wide stance to the start position, lowering your arms as you go.

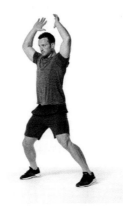 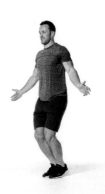

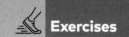

Stretch away stress

Take some time after exercise to stretch your muscles for improved mobility!

Warming up before a workout is really important, and so is taking a little time after your session to let your body readjust back to a resting state from a highly active one. Stretching is a fantastic way to help your body return to its natural state, and a great way to improve your mobility and flexibility. Over the next three pages we detail eight stretches to do after your workout, and remember – don't hold your breath when stretching! This is easy to do because stretching can sometimes be uncomfortable, but forgetting to breathe will stress your body and send your heart rate and blood pressure soaring, which is the opposite of what you're aiming for. Keep your breathing deep, slow and controlled to lower your heart rate, and breathe out through pursed lips when taking your stretches a little bit deeper.

Chest

- Kneel down and interlink your fingers behind your back. Keep your chest up and straighten your arms behind your back. Hold this position for 30 seconds.

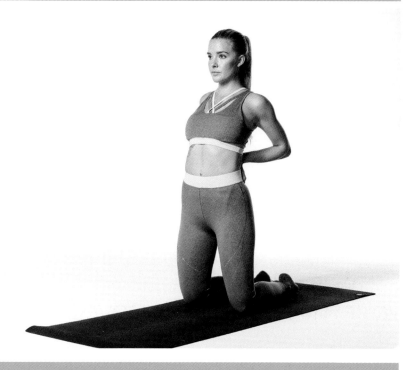

Triceps

- Put one hand back behind your back and the other behind your head, then interlock your fingers. Keep your chest up and pull as if trying to pull your hands away from each other. Hold this position for 30 seconds, then switch arms and repeat.

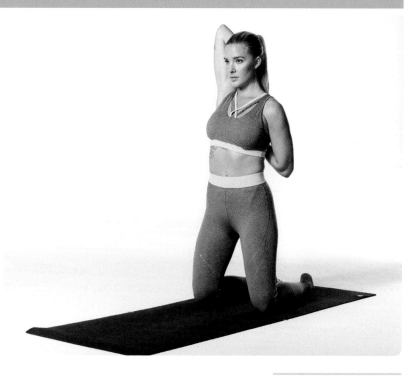

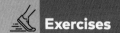
Back

- Kneel down, then lean forwards with straight arms. Keeping your head down, reach as far forwards as you can until you feel a good stretch across your back. Hold this position for 30 seconds.

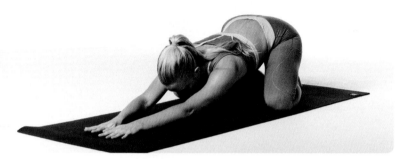

Lats (side back)

- Start on one knee with your other foot forward. Keeping your chest up, raise one arm above your head and lean over to one side. Hold this position for 30 seconds, then switch knees and arms and repeat.

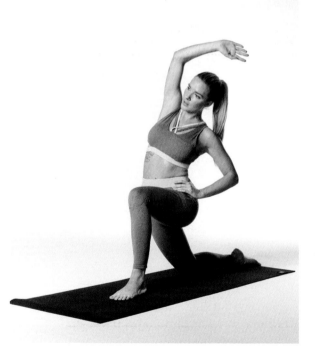

Hips

- Start on one knee with your other foot forward. Keeping your chest up, raise both arms above your head. Push your hips forwards until you feel a good stretch. Hold this position for 30 seconds, then switch knees and repeat.

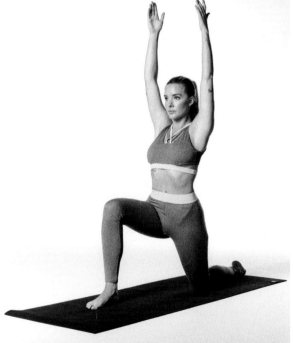

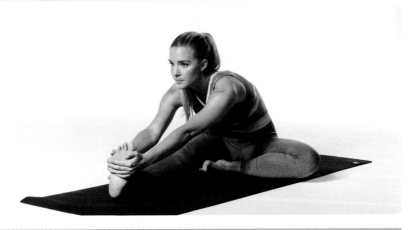

Hamstrings (back of thighs)

- Sit up with one leg straight out in front of you and your other leg bent with your foot against your straight leg. Lean forwards and reach down the front of your leg as far as you can. Hold this position for 30 seconds, then switch legs and repeat.

Quads (front of thighs)

- Lie on one side then bring the heel of your top leg towards your bum. Use your top hand to hold your foot and pull it further towards you to increase the stretch. Hold this position for 30 seconds, then switch legs and repeat.

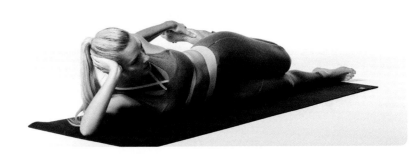

Glutes (bum)

- Lie on your back and bring one knee up. Bend your other leg and place that foot against your thigh. Loop your hands around your lower leg and pull it in towards you to increase the stretch. Hold this position for 30 seconds, then switch legs and repeat.

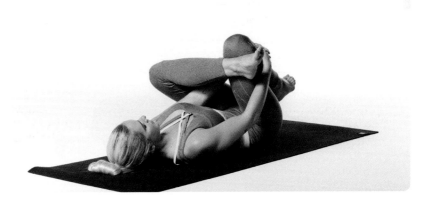

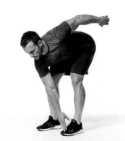
Alternating toe touch

- Stand tall with your chest up.
- Bend down from your hips, with a slight bend in your knees, and touch your right foot with your left hand.
- Stand back up and repeat, touching your left foot with your right hand.
- Alternate sides with each rep.

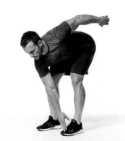
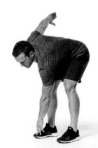

Arch hold

- Lie flat on your front with your core engaged and your arms straight out in front of you.
- Keeping your arms and legs straight, raise your hands and feet off the floor.
- Keep your abs and glutes (bum muscles) engaged to hold this position.
- Keep your breathing controlled and relaxed.

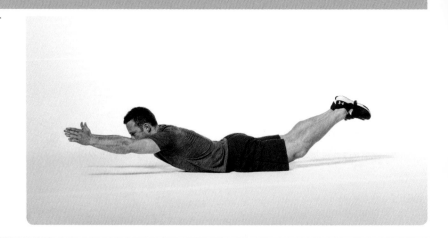

Bear crawl

- Start on all fours with your palms and toes on the floor and your knees underneath your body.
- Keep your back straight and your abs engaged.
- Make short and quick movements with opposite hands and feet to "crawl" forwards.
- If you're short of space simply do a few movements forwards then a few backwards, and repeat.

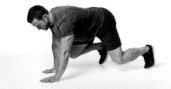
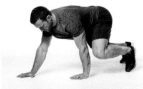

Bicycle

- Lie flat on your back with your fingers by your temples and legs straight.

- Raise your torso off the floor, engage your abs, and lift your feet off the floor.

- Crunch up and rotate your torso to one side, bringing your opposite knee in to touch your elbow.

- Reverse the movement to return to the starting position (without your upper back or feet touching the floor), then repeat on the other side.

- Alternate sides with each rep.

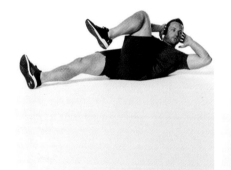 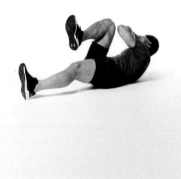

Bulgarian split squat

- Stand tall on one leg with your other foot placed on a chair or raised surface behind you.

- Keeping your chest up and abs engaged, bend your front knee to lower as far as you can.

- Push back off your front foot to return to the start position.

- Halfway through the set, change legs.

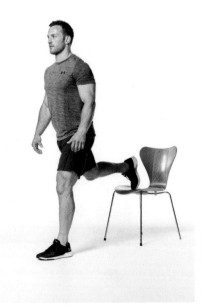 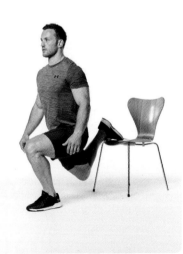

Burpee

- Stand tall with your chest up and arms by your sides.
- Drop down so your palms are on the floor with your knees by your chest.
- Kick your legs out so your body forms a straight line from head to heels.
- Bring your knees back under your body, then jump up into the air.
- As you land, go straight into the next rep.

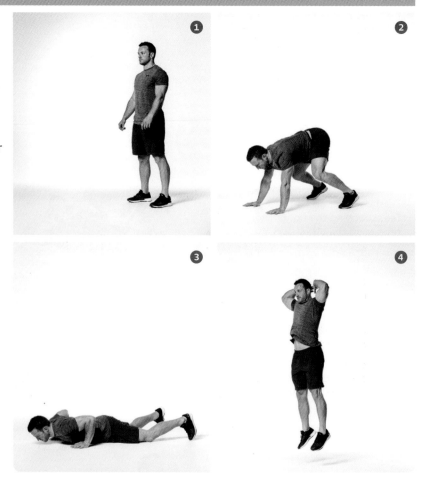

Butt kick

- Stand tall with your chest up and abs engaged.
- Kick one foot up behind you so your heel touches your bum, then return it to the floor and kick the other up.
- Remain on the same spot, and don't move forwards or backwards.
- Keep each butt kick fast but controlled, with your abs engaged throughout.

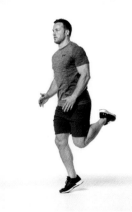
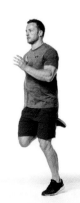

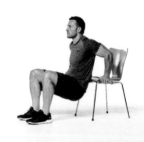

Chair dip bent knees

- Place your hands on the edge of a chair behind you with your arms straight and knees bent.

- Keeping your chest up, bend your elbows to lower your bum towards the floor.

- Go as low as you can, then press back up to straighten your arms and return to the start position.

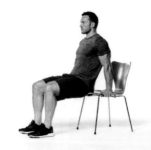

Chair dip straight legs

- Place your hands on the edge of a chair behind you with your arms straight and legs straight.

- Keeping your chest up, bend your elbows to lower your bum towards the floor.

- Go as low as you can, then press back up to straighten your arms and return to the start position.

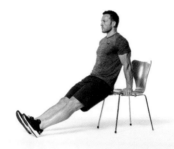
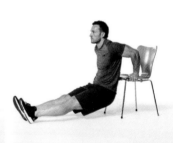

Chair press-up

- Place your hands on the seat of a chair in front of you with straight arms and your body straight from head to heels.

- Engage your abs and bend your elbows to lower your chest towards the seat.

- Go as low as you can, then press back up to straighten your arms and return to the start position.

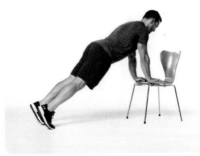
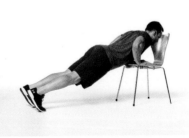

Chair squat

- Stand tall with a chair behind you.

- Keeping your chest up and abs engaged, bend your knees to squat down and raise your arms in front of you to shoulder height.

- Once your bum touches the chair, straighten your legs and stand back up to return to the start position.

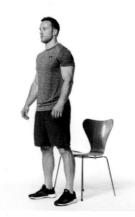 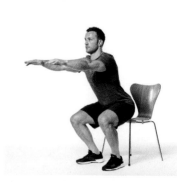

Crunch

- Lie flat on your back with your knees bent and feet flat on the floor, and bend your arms so your fingers touch the side of your head.

- Engage your abs, then raise your torso off the floor without tensing your neck.

- Keep that tension on your abs as you slowly lower your torso back to the floor.

- Make the move harder by not allowing your upper back to touch the floor between reps.

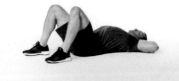 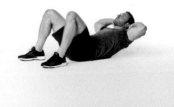

Curtsy lunge

- Stand tall with your chest up, your abs engaged and your hands by your sides.

- Keeping your chest up place one foot behind the other, then bend both knees to lunge down until your back knee almost touches the floor.

- Push off your rear foot to return to the start position, then repeat, leading with your other leg. Alternate legs with each rep.

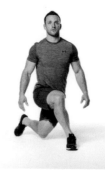 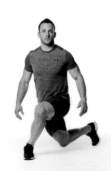

Diagonal mountain climber

- Get on all fours with your arms and legs straight and your wrists directly under your shoulders.

- Without letting your hips sag, draw one knee in and bring it across towards the opposite elbow.

- Straighten that leg then repeat, bringing your other knee towards its opposite elbow.

- Keep your abs engaged throughout and keep the reps fast but controlled.

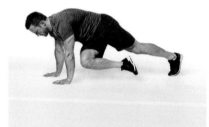 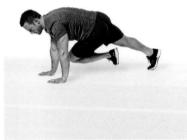

Down-up

- Stand tall with your chest up and arms by your sides.

- Drop down so your palms are on the floor with your knees by your chest.

- Kick your legs out so your body forms a straight line from head to heels.

- Bring your knees back under your body, then stand back up.

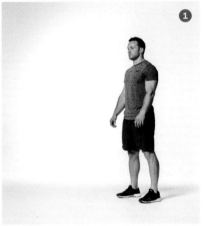 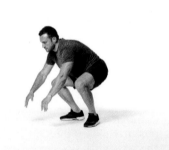

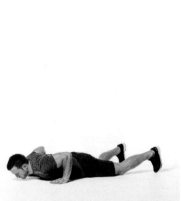 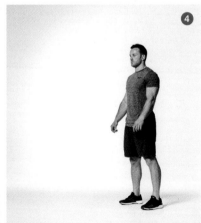

Glute bridge

- Lie flat on your back with your hands on your stomach and your knees bent.

- Engage your abs and your glutes (bum muscles), then raise your hips off the floor.

- Squeeze your glutes hard at the top, then lower your hips to return to the start position.

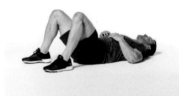
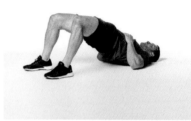

Half Turkish get-up

- Lie flat on your back with your right arm raised and straight and your right leg bent. Your left arm should be straight and out to the side.

- Raise your upper body off the floor by straightening your left arm, keeping your right arm straight and directly overhead.

- Lift your hips off the floor by pushing down through your right foot, then hold this position.

- Return to the start and repeat. Halfway through the set, switch sides.

1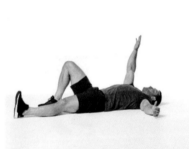

2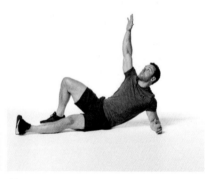

3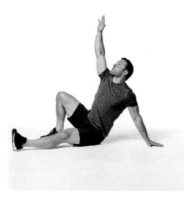

4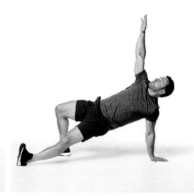

Hands-up press-up

- Get into a press-up position with your legs and arms straight and your palms flat on the floor.

- Engage your abs, then bend your elbows to lower your chest to the floor.

- Once your chest is on the floor, lift your palms up and off the floor.

- Return your palms to the floor, then press back up to straighten your arms and return to the start position.

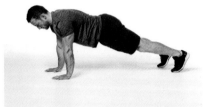 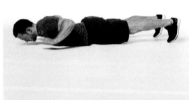

Heel touch

- Lie flat on your back with your knees bent and arms straight and by your sides.

- Keeping your arms straight, engage your abs and reach down with your left hand to tap your left heel, then your right hand to tap your right heel. Keep alternating.

- Keep your breathing controlled and relaxed.

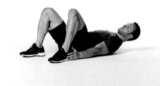 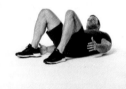

High knees

- Stand tall with your chest up and abs engaged.

- Start sprinting on the spot, swinging your arms and bringing your knees up as high as possible.

- You can also put your arms out straight in front of you and try to make your knees hit your palms with each step.

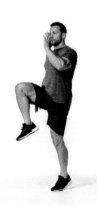 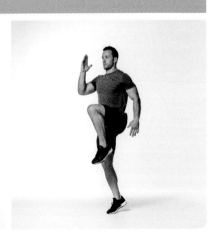

Hollow body

- Lie flat on your back with legs straight and arms straight behind you.

- Raise your arms and legs so that your body forms a bowl shape.

- Hold this position, keeping your breathing controlled.

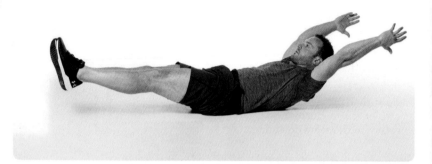

Jackknife

- Lie flat on your back with your legs straight and your arms straight and pointing above your head. Engage your abs.

- Keeping your arms and legs straight, raise your arms and feet off the floor, and bring your arms forwards so your hands touch your legs.

- Try and reach as far up your leg as possible to work your abs harder.

- Reverse the movement to return to the start position.

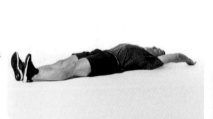
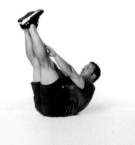

Lateral bear crawl

- Start on all fours with your palms and toes on the floor and your knees underneath your body.

- Keep your back straight and your abs engaged.

- Make short and quick movements with opposite hands and feet to "crawl" to one side.

- If you're short of space simply do a few movements sideways, then back again, and repeat.

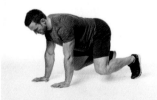
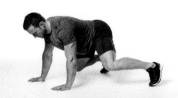

Lateral jump

- Stand tall with your chest up and your arms by your sides.

- Bend your knees slightly, then jump up and across to one side, swinging your arms for momentum.

- Land on both feet, then go straight into the next jump, jumping back the other way.

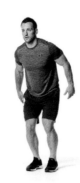 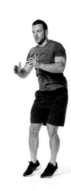

Lateral press-up

- Get on all fours with your legs and arms straight and with your hands under your shoulders.

- Engage your abs and bring your left hand out to the side, then bend both elbows to lower your chest down to the floor.

- Press back up to the start, then bring your left hand back underneath your shoulder. Take your right hand out to the side and repeat the move. Alternate which hand moves to the side with each rep.

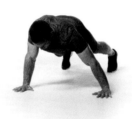 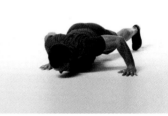

Lateral squat

- Stand tall with your feet wide apart and your chest up.

- Engage your abs, then bend your left knee to lower your bum towards the floor, keeping your right leg straight.

- Push through your left foot to return to the start position, then repeat the move, bending your right knee and lowering to that side.

- Alternate sides with each rep.

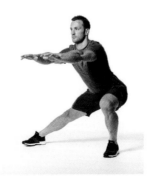 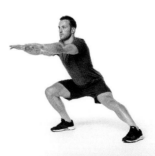

Lean-over lunge

- Stand tall with your chest up, abs engaged and arms raised straight above your head.

- Take a big step forwards with your left foot and bend both knees to lunge down while leaning over to your left.

- Push through your front foot to return to the start, then step forwards with your right foot and repeat the move, leaning to your right.

- Alternate sides with each rep.

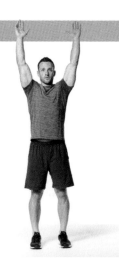 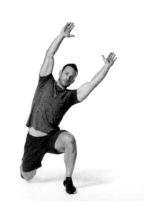

Lean-over reverse lunge

- Stand tall with your chest up, abs engaged and arms raised straight above your head.

- Take a big step backwards with your right foot and bend both knees to lunge down while leaning over to your left.

- Push through your back foot to return to the start, then step backwards with your left foot and repeat the move, leaning to your right.

- Alternate sides with each rep.

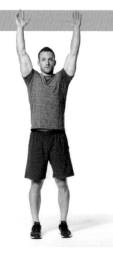 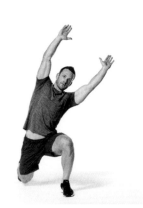

Leg raise

- Lie flat on your back with your legs straight and hands across your stomach or under the small of your back.

- Engage your abs, then raise your feet off the floor.

- Keeping your legs straight, raise your feet as high as you can, then slowly lower them.

- You can make the move harder and work your lower abs more by not allowing your heels to touch the floor between reps.

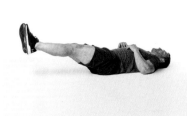 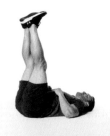

Leg raise hold

- Lie flat on your back with your legs straight and hands across your stomach or under the small of your back.

- Engage your abs, then raise your feet off the floor.

- Keeping your legs straight, raise your feet as high as you can.

- Keep your abs fully engaged to hold this position, keeping your breathing controlled.

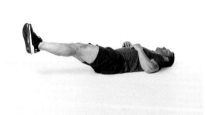
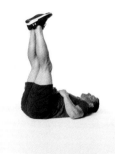

Lunge

- Stand tall with your chest up and abs engaged.

- Take a big step forwards with your left foot, then bend both knees to lunge down until your knees almost touch the floor.

- Push through your front foot to return to the start, then step forwards with your right foot and repeat the move.

- Alternate sides with each rep.

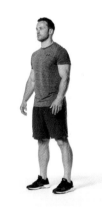
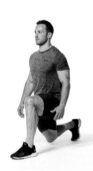

Lunge with arm raise

- Stand tall with your chest up, abs engaged and arms by your sides.

- Take a big step forwards with your left foot, then bend both knees to lunge down, while raising your arms directly overhead.

- Push through your front foot to return to the start, then step forwards with your right foot and repeat the move.

- Alternate sides with each rep.

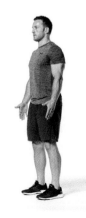
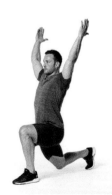

Marching glute bridge

- Lie flat on your back with your hands on your chest and your knees bent.

- Engage your abs and your glutes (bum muscles), then raise your hips off the floor.

- Straighten your left leg to raise your left foot off the floor.

- Return your left foot to the floor, then straighten your right leg to raise your right foot off the floor.

- Alternate legs with each rep.

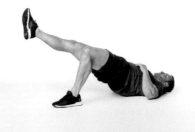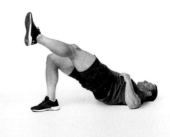

Mountain climber

- Get on all fours with your arms and legs straight and your wrists directly under your shoulders.

- Without letting your hips sag, draw one knee up and bring it towards the elbow on the same side.

- Straighten that leg, then repeat, bringing your other knee towards your elbow.

- Keep your abs engaged throughout and keep the reps fast but controlled.

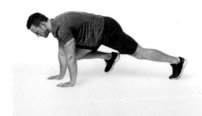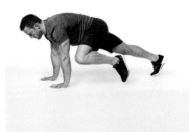

Offset press-up

- Get on all fours with your legs and arms straight with your hands under your shoulders.

- Engage your abs and move your right hand out in front of you, then bend both elbows to lower your chest to the floor.

- Press back up to the start, then bring your right hand back underneath your shoulder. Move your left hand out in front of you and repeat the move.

- Alternate sides with each rep.

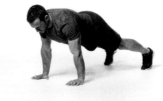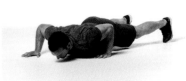

Overhead reverse lunge

- Stand tall with your chest up, abs engaged and arms raised directly overhead.
- Take a big step backwards with your right foot, then bend both knees to lunge down, keeping your arms overhead.
- Push through your back foot to return to the start, then step backwards with your left foot and repeat the move.
- Alternate sides with each rep.

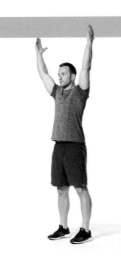
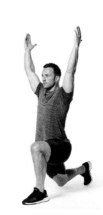

Overhead squat

- Stand tall with your chest up, abs engaged and arms raised directly overhead.
- Bend your knees to squat down as low as you can, keeping your arms straight overhead.
- Push through your heels to straighten your legs and return to the start position.

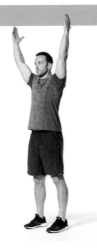
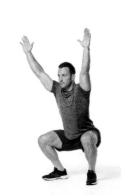

Pause squat

- Stand tall with your chest up, abs engaged and arms by your sides.
- Bend your knees to squat down as low as you can, bringing your arms out in front of you to shoulder height.
- Keep your chest up and abs engaged and maintain this position. If you start to struggle, stand back up, take two deep breaths, then squat back down and hold.

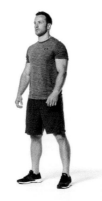
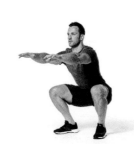

Pike

- Get on all fours with your arms and legs straight and your wrists directly under your shoulders.

- Keeping your abs engaged, raise your hips as high as you can so you go up onto your tiptoes.

- Lower your hips to return to the start.

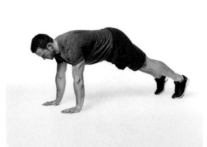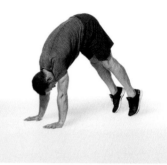

Plank

- Get into position, supporting yourself on your forearms with your elbows underneath your shoulders.

- Engage your abs, then raise your hips so that your body forms a straight line from head to heels.

- Hold this position by keeping your abs and glutes engaged to prevent your hips from sagging.

- Keep your breathing controlled and relaxed.

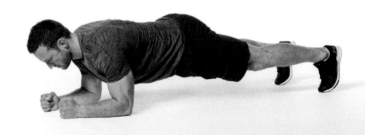

Plank jack

- Get into position, supporting yourself on your forearms with your elbows underneath your shoulders.

- Engage your abs, then raise your hips so that your body forms a straight line from head to heels.

- Without letting your hips sag, jump both feet out to the sides, then back in and continue repeating this movement.

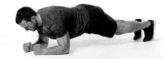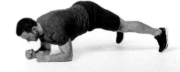

Pogo

- Stand tall with your chest up, abs engaged and arms by your sides.

- Spring straight up into the air, keeping your arms by your sides.

- Land on both feet and go straight into the next jump.

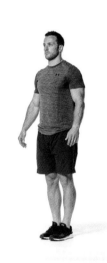
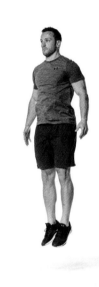

Press-up

- Get on all fours with your legs and arms straight, your hands under your shoulders and your body in a straight line from head to heels.

- Engage your abs and bend your elbows to lower your chest towards the floor.

- Go as low as you can, then press back up to straighten your arms and return to the start position.

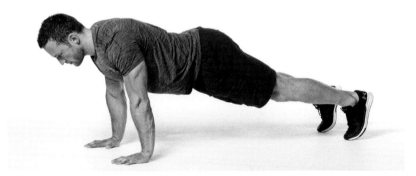

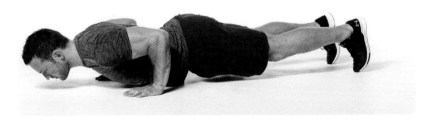

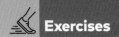
Press-up knees-up

- Get on all fours with your legs and arms straight, your hands under your shoulders and your body in a straight line from head to heels.

- Engage your abs and bend your elbows to lower your chest down towards the floor.

- Go as low as you can and let your knees touch the floor.

- Press back up to straighten your arms, and then go onto your toes to return to the start position.

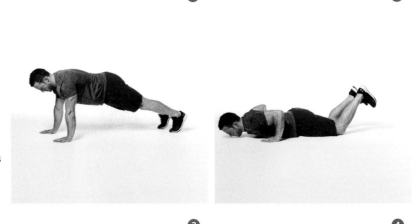

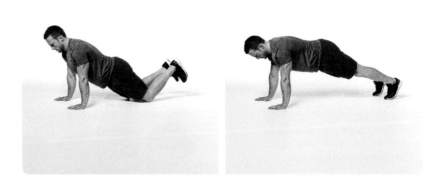

Prisoner lunge

- Stand tall with your chest up, abs engaged and elbows bent with your hands behind your head.

- Take a big step forwards with your right foot, then bend both knees to lunge down until your knees almost touch the floor.

- Push through your front foot to return to the start, then step forwards with your left foot and repeat the move.

- Alternate sides with each rep.

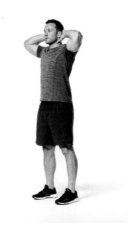

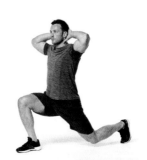

Prisoner squat

- Stand tall with your chest up, abs engaged and elbows bent with your hands behind your head

- Bend your knees to squat down as low as you can.

- Push through your heels to straighten your legs and return to the start position.

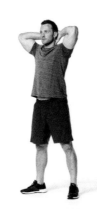 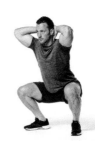

Reverse lunge

- Stand tall with your chest up and abs engaged.

- Take a big step backwards with your right foot, then bend both knees to lunge down until your knees almost touch the floor.

- Push through your back foot to return to the start, then step backwards with your left foot and repeat the move.

- Alternate sides with each rep.

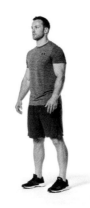 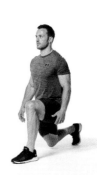

Rolling plank

- Get into position, supporting yourself on your forearms with your elbows underneath your shoulders.

- Engage your abs, then raise your hips off the floor so that your body forms a straight line from head to heels. Hold this position.

- Roll one side of your hips down towards the floor, then back to the top, then repeat on the other side. Continue alternating.

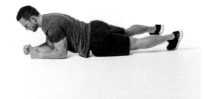 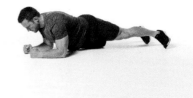

Romanian deadlift

- Stand tall with your chest up and abs engaged.

- With a slight bend in your knees, bend forwards from the hips and reach down the front of your legs, touching your fingertips to them as low down as possible.

- Stand up to return to the start position.

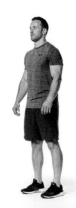 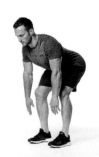

Rotating lunge

- Stand tall with your chest up, abs engaged and arms straight out in front of you.

- Take a big step forwards with your left foot, then bend both knees to lunge down while rotating your torso to your left.

- Push through your front foot and rotate back to the start, then step forwards with your right foot and repeat the move, rotating your torso to the right.

- Alternate sides with each rep.

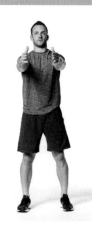 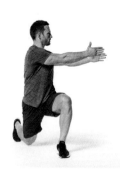

Rotating reverse lunge

- Stand tall with your chest up, abs engaged and arms straight out in front of you.

- Take a big step backwards with your left foot, then bend both knees to lunge down while rotating your torso to your right.

- Push through your back foot and rotate back to the start, then step backwards with your right foot and repeat the move, rotating your torso to the left.

- Alternate sides with each rep.

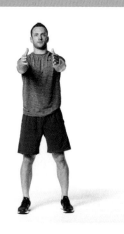 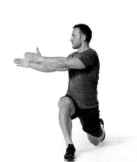

Seated Russian twist

- Sit up with your chest up, abs engaged and a slight bend in your knees.

- Use your abs to rotate your torso to one side, then return to the middle and rotate to the other side.

- Make the move harder by raising your heels off the floor and keeping them raised.

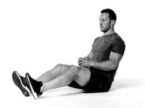 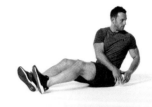

Side lunge

- Stand tall with your chest up, abs engaged and arms by your sides.

- Take a big step to your left, then bend your left leg to lunge down while raising your arms in front of you to shoulder height.

- Push through your left foot to return to the start, then repeat by taking a big step to your right.

- Alternate sides with each rep.

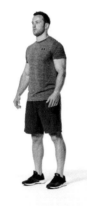 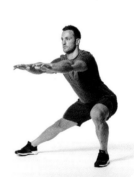

Side plank

- Lie on your side, supporting your upper body on your left forearm.

- Engage your abs, then raise your hips so that your body forms a straight line from head to heels.

- Keep your abs and glutes (bum muscles) engaged to hold this position without letting your hips sag.

- Keep your breathing controlled and relaxed.

- Halfway through the set, switch sides.

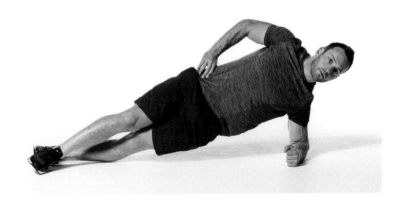

Single-leg glute bridge

- Lie flat on your back with your left leg bent and your right leg raised and straight.

- Engage your abs and your glutes (bum muscles), then raise your hips off the floor, keeping your left leg straight.

- Squeeze your glutes hard at the top, then lower your hips to return to the start position. Halfway through the set, change legs.

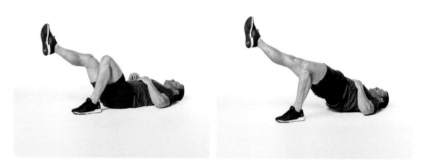

Single-leg hollow body

- Lie flat on your back with your right leg straight and your left knee drawn in towards your torso, and your arms pointing straight above your head.

- Raise your arms and your right leg so that your body forms a bowl shape.

- Hold this position, keeping your breathing controlled. Halfway through the set, change legs.

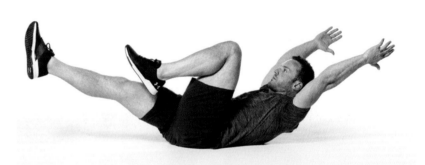

Single-leg Romanian deadlift

- Stand tall on your left leg with your chest up and abs engaged.

- With a slight bend in your left knee, bend forwards from the hips and reach down the front of your left leg, touching your fingertips to it as low down as possible.

- Return to the start position. Halfway through the set, change legs.

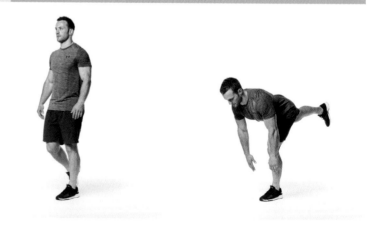

Single-leg Romanian deadlift reach

- Stand tall on your left leg with your chest up, abs engaged and arms straight out in front of you.

- With a slight bend in your left knee, bend forwards from the hips then reach your fingertips forwards as far as possible, raising your right leg behind you for balance.

- Return to the start position and repeat. Halfway through the set, change legs.

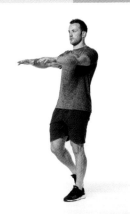
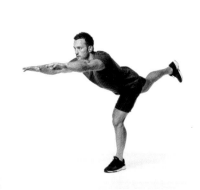

Single-leg Russian twist

- Sit up with your chest up, abs engaged and a slight bend in your left knee so it's higher than your right leg, which you should hold straight. Keep both heels off the floor.

- Use your abs to rotate your torso to one side, then return to the middle and rotate to the other side.

- Halfway through the set, change legs.

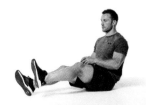
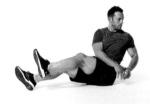

Speed skater

- Stand tall on one leg with your chest up and abs engaged.

- Leap up and across to land on your other leg, swinging your arms for momentum. Your non-standing foot should go behind your standing leg.

- As soon as you land on your other foot leap straight back into the next rep, keeping your movements fast but controlled.

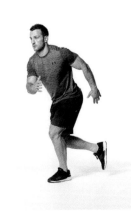
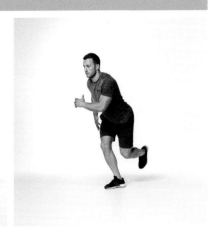

Spider-Man press-up

- Start with your palms on the floor, your wrists underneath your shoulders and your body in a straight line from head to heels.

- Engage your abs and bend your elbows to lower your chest towards the floor. As you do, bring one knee up so that it touches your arm.

- Press back up to straighten your arms and return to the start position. Repeat, bringing in the other knee, and alternate sides with each rep.

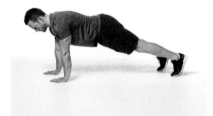
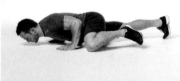

Split squat

- Stand tall with one foot forward and your chest up and abs engaged.

- Bend both knees to lower until your knee almost touches the floor.

- Push through your front foot to return to the start and repeat. Halfway through the set change legs.

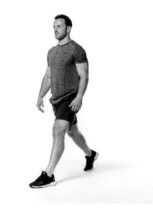
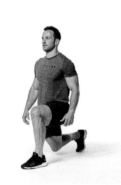

Squat

- Stand tall with your chest up, abs engaged and arms straight by your sides.

- Bend your knees to squat down as low as you can, either keeping your arms by your sides or raising them up to shoulder height.

- Push through your heels to straighten your legs and return to the start position.

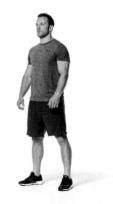
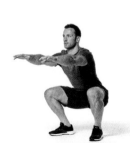

Squat hold

- Stand tall with your chest up, abs engaged and arms straight by your sides.

- Bend your knees to squat down as low as you can while bringing your arms out in front of you to shoulder height.

- Keeping your chest up and abs engaged, maintain this position. If you start to struggle, straighten your legs a little so you're not as deep, then hold that position.

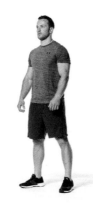
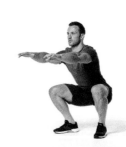

Squat jump

- Stand tall with your chest up, abs engaged and arms straight by your sides.

- Bend your knees to squat down as low as you can, and swing your arms backwards.

- Push through your heels to straighten your legs and jump powerfully off the floor.

- Land on both feet and go straight into the next rep.

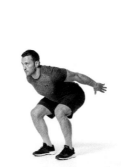
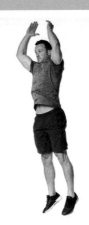

Squat thrust

- Start with your palms on the floor with your wrists underneath your shoulders and your body in a straight line from head to heels.

- Keeping your back straight and your abs engaged, draw your knees in towards your chest so that both feet land under your body.

- Jump your feet back out to straighten your legs.

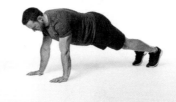
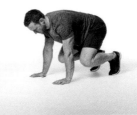

Standing jog

- Stand tall with your chest up and abs engaged.

- Jog on the spot, swinging your arms back and forth.

- Make this move more effective by alternating short bursts of faster jogging with slower jogging.

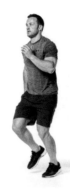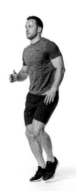

Standing Russian twist

- Stand tall with your chest up and abs engaged, with your arms out straight in front of you and hands clasped together.

- Keeping your hips facing forwards, rotate your torso all the way to one side and then back across to the other.

- Keep the reps fast but controlled, with your abs engaged throughout.

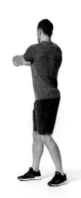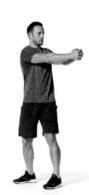

Standing sprint

- Stand tall with your chest up and abs engaged.

- Sprint on the spot, raising your knees as high as possible and swinging your arms back and forth.

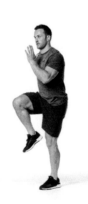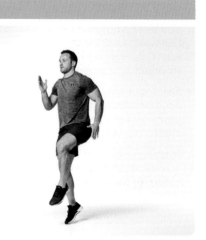

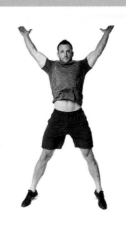

Star jump

- Stand tall with your chest up, abs engaged and hands by your sides.

- Jump up and bring both feet out wide to the sides while raising your arms to the sides so your hands finish above your head.

- Jump back from the wide stance to the start position, lowering your arms as you go.

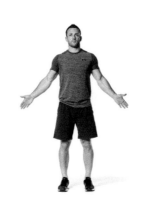

Static bear crawl

- Get on all fours with your palms and toes on the floor and your knees underneath your body.

- Keep your back straight and your abs engaged.

- Move your left hand and right foot forward, touch the floor, then bring them back, then repeat, moving your right hand and left foot forward. Continue alternating.

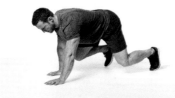 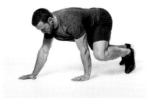

Sumo squat

- Stand tall with your feet double hip-width apart with your chest up, abs engaged and arms straight by your sides.

- Bend your knees to squat down as low as you can, either keeping your arms by your sides or raising them up to shoulder height.

- Push through your heels to straighten your legs and return to the start position.

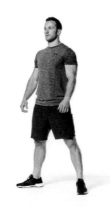 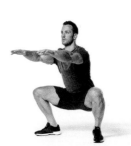

T press-up

- Get into position with your palms on the floor, your wrists underneath your shoulders and your body in a straight line from head to heels.

- Engage your abs and bend your elbows to lower your chest down towards the floor.

- Go as low as you can, then press back up. As you do, rotate your torso to raise one arm straight up.

- Lower it and go straight into the next rep, turning the other way and raising your other arm. Alternate sides with each rep.

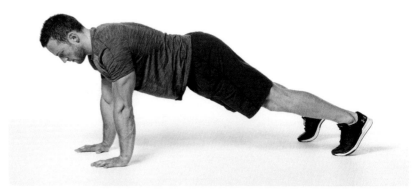

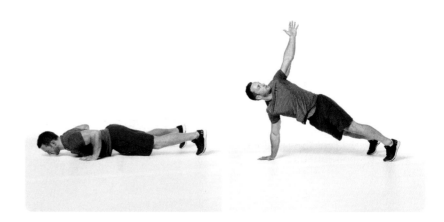

Tall plank

- Get into position with your palms on the floor, your wrists underneath your shoulders and your body in a straight line from head to heels.

- Keep your abs and glutes (bum muscles) engaged to hold this position without letting your hips sag.

- Keep your breathing controlled and relaxed.

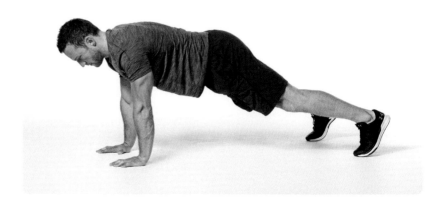

Tall plank shoulder tap

- Get into position with your palms on the floor, your wrists underneath your shoulders and your body in a straight line from head to heels.

- Keep your abs and glutes engaged to hold this position without letting your hips sag.

- Lift one hand off the floor and tap your opposite shoulder. Return it and repeat with your other hand.

- Keep your breathing controlled and relaxed.

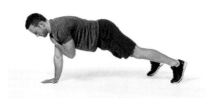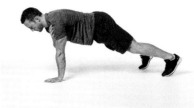

Tall plank toe tap

- Get into position with your palms on the floor, your wrists underneath your shoulders and your body in a straight line from head to heels.

- Keep your abs and glutes engaged to hold this position without letting your hips sag.

- Lift one foot off the floor and move it to the side. Tap the floor with your toes then return to the start. Repeat on the other side.

- Continue, alternating toe taps.

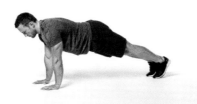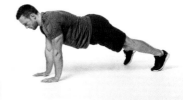

Tall side plank

- Lie on your side, supporting your upper body on your left hand.

- Engage your abs, then raise your hips so that your body forms a straight line from head to heels.

- Keep your abs and glutes engaged to hold this position without letting your hips sag. Halfway through the set, switch sides.

- Keep your breathing controlled and relaxed.

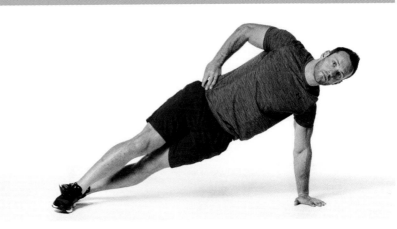

Turkish get-up

- Lie flat on your back with your left arm straight and raised straight up and your left leg bent. Your right arm should be straight and out to the side.

- Raise your upper body off the floor by straightening your left arm, keeping your left arm straight and directly overhead.

- Lift your hips off the floor by pushing down through your right, then bring your right foot in and underneath your body.

- Push down through your left heel to stand up straight, with your arm still overhead.

- Reverse the movement back to the start position and repeat. Halfway through the set, switch sides.

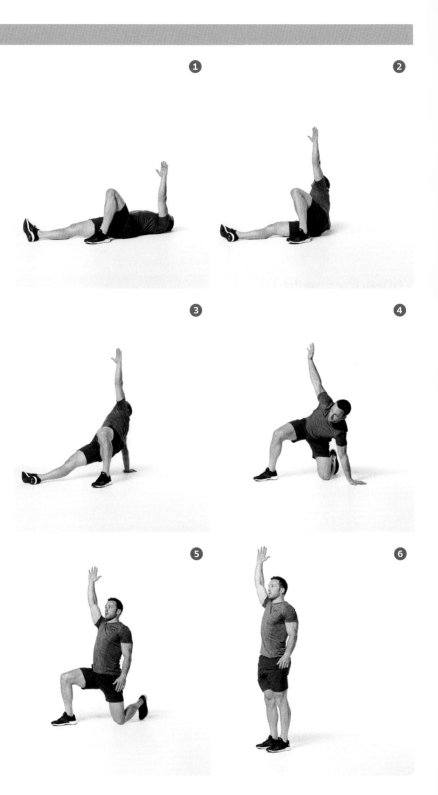

1 **2** **3** **4** **5** **6**

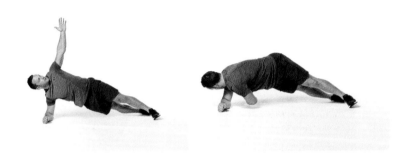

Thread the needle

- Get into position, supporting yourself on your forearms with your elbows underneath your shoulders.

- Lift one hand off the floor. Rotate your torso and raise that arm.

- Rotate back down and move that arm underneath your body, then rotate back again.

- Halfway through the set, switch sides.

Three-pulse squat

- Stand tall with your chest up, abs engaged and arms straight by your sides.

- Bend your knees to squat down as low as you can, either keeping your arms by your sides or raising them to shoulder height.

- In the bottom position of the squat, "pulse" up and down three times, then straighten your legs to return to the start position.

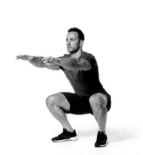
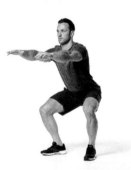

Transverse lunge

- Stand tall with your chest up, abs engaged and arms straight by your sides.

- Imagine your right foot is pointing to 12 on a clock face. Move your left foot back and plant it to point to 7.

- Bend both knees to lunge down, then push back off your back foot to return to the start.

- Repeat on the other leg, planting it to point to 5. Continue, alternating sides with each rep.

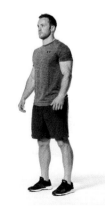
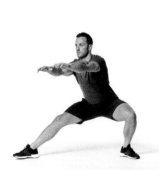

Tuck jump

- Stand tall with your chest up, abs engaged and arms straight by your sides.

- Bend your knees slightly, then jump up off the floor, raising your knees as high as you can.

- Land on both feet and go straight into the next rep.

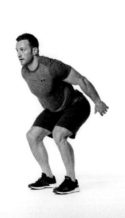
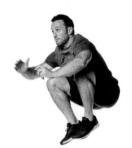

Two-pulse squat

- Stand tall with your chest up, abs engaged and arms straight by your sides.

- Bend your knees to squat down as low as you can, either keeping your arms by your sides or raising them to shoulder height.

- In the bottom position of the squat, "pulse" up and down twice, then straighten your legs to return to the start position.

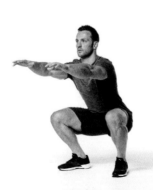
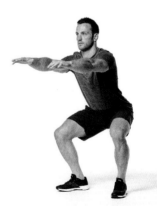

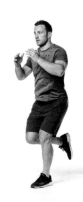

Two-to-one jump

- Stand tall with your chest up and your arms by your sides.

- Bend your knees slightly then jump up and across to one side, swinging your arms for momentum, and land on one foot.

- Go straight into the next jump, jumping back across to land on two feet. Then repeat the move but jump in the other direction to land on one foot, then jump back.

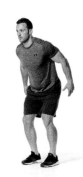

Walking down-up

- Stand tall with your chest up and your arms by your sides.

- Drop down onto your hands and walk your feet back behind you so you're lying flat on the floor.

- Press your torso back up and walk your feet back in to bring your knees in and underneath you, then stand back up.

1   **2**

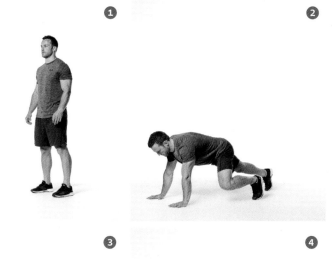

3   **4**

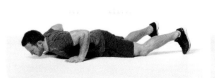 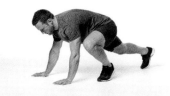

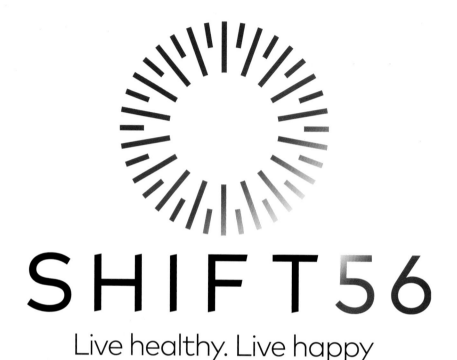

SHIFT56

Live healthy. Live happy

We'd love to hear about your SHIFT56 journey towards a leaner, healthier and happier life. Share your story with us using #shift56!

@Shift_56

@Shift56

@TheShift56System